Praise for

MIDLIFE UPGRADE

"Honest and empowering. More people deserve to know what is coming in midlife. This book delivers!"

—Kelly Casperson, MD,
bestselling author of *You Are Not Broken* and the award-winning podcast by the same name
INSTAGRAM / @kellycaspersonmd

"*Midlife Upgrade* isn't just a guide—it's a lifeline for any woman navigating the chaos and beauty of midlife. Julie and Pam have done what so many women dream of: they've turned honest conversations between best friends into a compassionate, evidence-based, and empowering manual for this next chapter. Whether you're facing hot flashes, brain fog, or just the need to feel seen, these pages deliver wisdom, warmth, and real solutions—with a sense of humor and a fierce belief in your power to thrive."

—Tamsen Fadal,
The New York Times bestselling author of *How to Menopause* and documentary producer of *The (M) Factor*
INSTAGRAM / @tamsenfadal

"Congratulations to Julie and Pamela on the publication of your insightful book, *Midlife Upgrade*! This thoughtful exploration beautifully captures the complexities and joys of midlife. Your work will inspire many to embrace this transformative phase with confidence and grace. Well done!"

—Dr. Sharon Malone,
Chief Medical Advisor, Alloy Women's Health,
The New York Times bestselling author of *Grown Woman Talk*
INSTAGRAM / @smalonemd

"Midlife isn't the beginning of the end; it's the beginning of ownership. This book is a wake-up call wrapped in wisdom. Julie and Pamela don't sugarcoat the symptoms or sidestep the stigma; they confront the silence around menopause, identity shifts, loss, and reinvention with honesty, elegance, and experience. This book doesn't ask women to cope, it challenges them to upgrade. If you've ever been told 'this is just part of getting older,' this book is for YOU!"

—Somi Javaid, MD, FACOG,
founder, HerMD, and disruptHER podcast,
INSTAGRAM / @somijavaidmd

"How completely apropos and timely to read a book by two best friends who discover and nurture each other and their surrounding hive through menopause and yet how shocking that this has not yet been done given the fact that this is how life typically works and works at its best—by listening and learning and an exchange of energy between two people with a shared experience! Who better to guide you through the shite that is perimenopause into the post-menopausal years than your BFF? Kudos to Pam and Julie for documenting the journey that SO many women traverse—the lucky ones have their best gal pals (and a handful of great clinicians) by their side. For the rest, there's *Midlife Upgrade!*"

—SHIEVA GHOFRANY, MD, OBGYN,
co-founder of Tribe Called V
INSTAGRAM/@drshievag

"Julie and Pam's contribution to the modern experience of the menopause transition is so very welcome. The groundswell of interest in this critical time in our lives has led to a lot of discussion and also a lot of confusion. What is really going on? What sources of advice are legitimate and vetted? This outstanding guide comes from the perspective of 'regular folks' and is supported by readily understood evidence and expert opinion. One size will never fit all. Just as *Menopause Bootcamp* supports agency via education and community, *Midlife Upgrade* creates another opportunity for us to evolve our perspective together."

—SUZANNE GILBERG-LENZ, MD, FACOG,
bestselling author of *Menopause Bootcamp*
INSTAGRAM/@askdrsuzanne

"Julie and Pam have written the guide every midlife woman deserves but never knew she needed. With a perfect blend of humor, spunk, and heartfelt honesty, they tackle the highs, lows, and WTF moments of menopause and beyond. This isn't just a book—it's a rallying cry for women to embrace their power, rewrite the rules, and navigate midlife on their own terms. Candid, compassionate, and full of real-life wisdom, it's like having your two best friends walk with you through your best chapter yet."

—SAMEENA RAHMAN, MD,
specialist in menopause care
INSTAGRAM/@gynogirl

"*Midlife Upgrade* is a poignant and thought-provoking exploration of midlife, offering a refreshing blend of personal stories, humor, and insight. Reading it feels like curling up on the couch with your best friend, a warm cup of coffee in hand, ready for heartfelt stories that resonate deeply with your own experiences. The book provides a voice that is both empowering and comforting, acting as a powerhouse of guidance. Much like the beloved classics we read during adolescence, this book is a modern-day companion—familiar, transformative, and full of wisdom for the road ahead. It's exactly what you need to feel seen, supported, and ready for what comes next. This is the book for you and all of your girlfriends!"

—CHRISTINE HART KRESS, DNP, MSCP
INSTAGRAM/@christinehartkress_dnp

"This insightful and accessible guide, written by two best friends who bonded through their own menopause journeys, is a much-needed resource for women navigating this transition. Recognizing the gap in both public and medical knowledge, they've created a book that demystifies perimenopause and menopause, combining holistic care approaches with evidence-based Western medicine. Whether you're considering hormone therapy or seeking non-hormonal options, this book respects and supports every choice, empowering women with knowledge and encouraging them to take charge of their health. A must-read for anyone looking for compassionate, comprehensive, and practical menopause guidance."

—AOIFE O'SULLIVAN MD, MSCP
INSTAGRAM/@portlandmenopausedoc

"No one prepares us for the chaos that hits in perimenopause. So who is it that women first turn to in order to figure out what the hell is happening to their bodies and brains? It is not their doctor; it is their BFFs! If you don't have best friends who can help you through this chaos that is 'ovarian retirement' and point you toward some reliable solutions or just reassure you that you are not losing your mind, you have Julie and Pam. They are two real-life BFFs who rode this crazy ride together. They are determined to help women navigate the path to restoring their mental and physical health with evidence-based advice and claiming their voice in self-advocacy. Read this and share it with your BFF or any midlife women you love."

—KATE WHITE, MD, FACOG, MSCP,
gynecologist, menopause and sexual health specialist
INSTAGRAM/@DrKateWhiteObGyn

"This menopause guidebook comes from the lens of midlife women who come together to bring perspective to a normal transition. During the menopause transition, women often feel unseen and unheard, and this guidebook is supported by readily understood evidence-based information as well as expert opinion in a manner that is easily digestible and relatable."

—HEATHER QUAILE, DNP, MSCP,
founder of The SHOW Center, founder and co-host of *justASK Podcast*
INSTAGRAM/@drquailenp

"Honest and empowering; deeply relatable. Julie and Pam bring humor, raw vulnerability, and a wealth of experiences that speak to the real struggles of midlife women. Their candid approach and evidence-backed guidance are a breath of fresh air in a world where menopause is often dismissed or misunderstood. This book isn't just informative—it's a testament to the strength and solidarity of women."

—Jackie Piasta,
women's health NP, co-host of *justASK Podcast*
instagram/@jackiep_gynnp

"*Midlife Upgrade* is an empowering guide that feels like a warm conversation with a trusted friend. With chapters on topics like sexual intimacy, personal freedom, and grief, it delves deeply into the emotional and physical aspects of menopause with honesty and grace. The authors strike a thoughtful balance, offering insights into not only coping but thriving. Practical advice on various diets, exercise routines, and supplements that have proven effective for the authors brings a refreshing, personalized touch to menopause symptom management. Uplifting and inclusive, this book is a supportive companion for every woman embracing midlife transformation."

—Rebbecca Hertel, DO, MSCP
instagram/@rebbeccaherteldo

"Julie Fedeli and Pamela DeRose are creating the solution they so needed when going through the menopausal transition. No woman should have to navigate this alone, yet most of us do. In *Midlife Upgrade*, they provide a girlfriend's guide on how to thrive through this powerful transition from a mind and body perspective."

—Dr. Laura Berman, PhD,
therapist, bestselling author, host of Language of Love podcast
instagram/@drlauraberman

MIDLIFE UPGRADE

A GIRLFRIEND'S GUIDE TO
FINDING YOUR POWER IN THE PAUSE

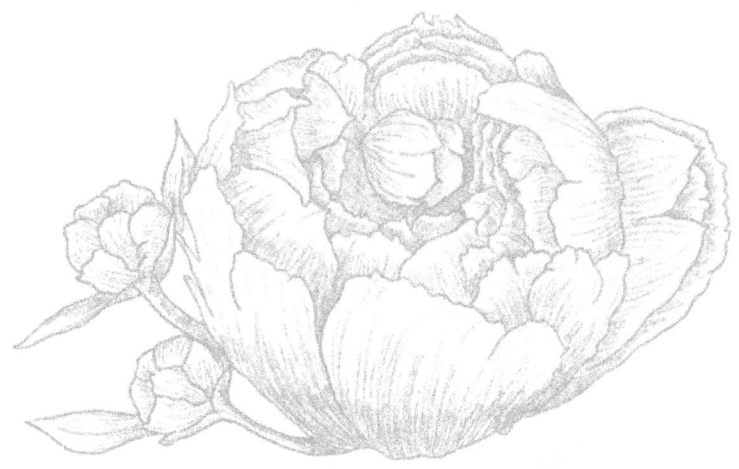

Julie Fedeli & Pamela DeRose

© 2025 Julie Fedeli and Pamela DeRose

Midlife Upgrade
A Girlfriend's Guide to Finding Your Power in the Pause

All rights reserved. No part of this publication may be reproduced, distributed, or transmitted in any form or by any means, including photocopying, recording, or other electronic or mechanical methods, without the prior written permission of the publisher, except in the case of brief quotations embodied in critical reviews and certain other noncommercial uses permitted by copyright law. For permission requests, write to the publisher, addressed "Attention: Permissions Coordinator," at the address below.

Published by
Thought Leader Academy
3901 North Kildare Avenue
Chicago, IL 60641

Library of Congress Control Number: 2025910693

ISBN: 979-8-9922574-1-0, 979-8-9922574-2-7 *(paperback)*
ISBN: 979-8-9922574-3-4 *(digital)*

HEALTH & FITNESS / Menopause
FAMILY & RELATIONSHIPS / Life Stages / Mid-Life
HEALTH & FITNESS / Women's Health
Printed in the United States of America

Cover design by Ram Fedeli
Interior book design by Claudine Mansour Design
Illustrations by Clara Baumgarten

We dedicate this book to our amazing friends,
clients, and all midlife women. May each of you always trust your
inner wisdom and know that you are truly invincible.

We are forever grateful for the
pioneering practitioners in the field of women's midlife health.
Keep fighting the good fight—we need you!

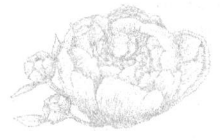

DISCLAIMER

The stories in this book are based on true events; however, names and certain details have been altered to safeguard the privacy of individuals. Every effort has been made to ensure the accuracy of the medical content provided in this book. However, it is essential to note that the authors are not medical professionals, and the information shared herein should not be construed as medical advice. Readers are encouraged to consult with their health care providers for personalized care tailored to their specific needs and circumstances.

The information in this book is for educational and entertainment purposes only. It is not intended to substitute professional medical, psychological, legal, financial, or other advice. The authors and publisher do not provide professional advice and expressly disclaim any responsibility for decisions made based on the content of this book.

This book is not intended to serve as the basis for any health, wellness, financial, or life-changing decisions. Readers are strongly encouraged to seek the guidance of qualified professionals, such as medical practitioners, financial advisors, or other experts, for advice specific to their situations.

The success stories, testimonials, and results shared in this book are for illustrative purposes only and do not represent typical outcomes. No guarantees are made regarding results or performance.

While every effort has been made to ensure the accuracy and completeness of the information provided, the authors and publisher make no representations, warranties, or guarantees, express or implied, regarding the content's accuracy, reliability, or completeness. The authors and publisher assume no responsibility or liability for any actions taken by readers as a result of the information in this book and expressly disclaim responsibility for any liability, loss, risk, or damage—whether physical, psychological, emotional, financial, or otherwise—that may arise directly or indirectly from the use or application of the content in this book.

Scan this code to access our exclusive BOOK PORTAL packed with powerful resources, inspiring playlists, guided meditations, and more. And don't stop there—you're also invited to join our Midlife Upgrade community and course, where real transformation and connection begins!

"People may call what happens at midlife 'a crisis.' But it's not. It's an unraveling—a time when you feel a desperate pull to live the life you want to live, not the one you're supposed to live. The unraveling is a time when you are challenged by the universe to let go of who you think you are supposed to be and embrace who you are."

—Brené Brown

CONTENTS

Authors' Note   xiv
Foreword   xv
Introduction   xvii

1. Peri-What?   1
2. Endocrine Harmony   18
3. It's Not Me. It's My Hormones!   37
4. Turn Yourself On   61
5. Self-Care Is the New Self-Care   85
6. Food to Live For   111
7. You Are Worthy   138
8. When Grief Arrives Midjourney   157
9. Together Stronger: Your Loving Relationships   183

Conclusion   205
Acknowledgments   209
Notes   212
Books We Recommend   229
About the Authors   233

AUTHORS' NOTE

You'll see the term HT used throughout this book. That stands for hormone therapy, which is sometimes also called HRT (hormone replacement therapy) or MHT (menopausal hormone therapy). The language keeps evolving, but most people still recognize HT, so that's what we're going with here.

Throughout this book, we use the words "woman," "women," and "female" to refer to people with ovaries. We recognize that not everyone who experiences menopause identifies with these terms, and language is evolving. Our intention is never to exclude—just to communicate clearly while holding space for everyone navigating this transition.

Let's be clear—menopause isn't just a "women's issue" in the traditional sense. While it's often framed around cisgender, heterosexual women, the reality is that many queer, nonbinary, and transgender people experience menopause too. And they often face even greater challenges when it comes to getting appropriate care, due to a serious lack of research, inclusive treatment options, and provider education. It's time we expand the conversation—and the care.

FOREWORD

—Jila Senemar, MD, FACOG-Instagram/@jilaamd

As a physician dedicated to women's health and menopause, I have had the privilege of guiding countless women through the complexities of midlife transitions. It is both an honor and a joy to write this foreword for *Midlife Upgrade*, a book that is as empowering as it is practical—a true game-changer for women seeking clarity, confidence, and renewal during one of life's most dynamic stages.

Julie Fedeli and Pamela DeRose have masterfully captured what so many women experience but rarely discuss: the surprises, struggles, and triumphs that accompany midlife. With wisdom rooted in lived experience and thoughtful research, they offer a guide that is not just informative but transformative. This is not merely a book; it is a lifeline for any woman who feels adrift in the sea of hormonal changes, emotional shifts, and new challenges that midlife can bring.

What I love most about *Midlife Upgrade* is its holistic approach. The authors tackle the physical and emotional realities of midlife, but they also go further, encouraging women to view this stage as an opportunity for transformation. From practical advice about sleep, nutrition, and hormonal health to candid discussions about relationships, sexuality, and personal growth, Julie and Pam provide a comprehensive toolkit for thriving—not just surviving—midlife.

In a world where the challenges of midlife are often dismissed or treated as something to endure, this book is a breath of fresh air. It breaks down complex topics in an accessible, friendly way that feels like having a trusted friend by your side. Julie and Pam share their personal stories with a candor and vulnerability that make their insights not only relatable but deeply validating. They remind us that we are not alone, that our experiences are valid, and that there is hope for a vibrant and fulfilling future.

This book is also a celebration of the resilience and wisdom that women bring to midlife. It challenges outdated narratives that suggest this season of life is a decline instead of championing the idea that it is an upgrade—a time to embrace change, rediscover purpose, and reclaim power. The authors' actionable strategies, coupled with inspiring anecdotes, make this book a treasure trove of support for women at any stage of their journey.

For me, the true beauty of *Midlife Upgrade* lies in its blend of practical guidance and heartfelt encouragement. It does not shy away from the challenges of midlife, but meets them head-on, offering tools and insights to help women navigate them with grace and strength. Whether you are struggling with hot flashes, seeking better sleep, grappling with shifts in your relationships, or simply longing for more joy in your daily life, this book will inspire you to take charge of your health and happiness.

As you read this book, I hope you will feel empowered to embrace the possibilities that lie ahead. With *Midlife Upgrade* in your hands, you have a powerful resource to guide you through this transformative stage of life. This is your time to shine, to prioritize yourself, and to live fully in ways that may have felt out of reach before.

To every woman reading this: You are not alone. Your experiences, challenges, and victories matter. Julie and Pam have created a resource that will meet you where you are and help guide you to where you want to be. I encourage you to dive in, embrace the journey, and know that your best years are still ahead.

INTRODUCTION

We have been friends for over a decade. Midlife friends are the best! We have navigated two children, three husbands, ten careers, and a lifetime of adventures. We have tried hundreds of supplements, explored numerous food plans, supported hundreds of clients and friends, shed millions of tears, and shared countless moments of laughter. Through it all, we have learned valuable lessons and discovered the secrets to living our best lives yet.

In May 2022, we got together for lunch and began talking about midlife sex! We shared things that we had *never* discussed before. And why not? Realizing that many conversations about the down and dirty of menopause were not happening, we decided to collaborate and create an amazing community program for midlife women. Holding that intention in our hearts, magical synchronicities began happening, and our *Midlife Upgrade* book was born.

We thought you might like to know a little more about us.

Pam

I became interested in health and nutrition when I was pregnant with my daughter 25 years ago. I knew I was only going to have one child, and I wanted to be the healthiest I could be. I read *Diet for a New America* by John Robbins, and it changed my life. I became a certified raw-food and vegan chef and attended the Institute for Integrative Nutrition, where I became a certified holistic health coach. I also spent some time learning about hormones and how they affect overall health. Knowing all that I do, one would think I'm super healthy and having the best midlife experience ever! Um, no.

Until the age of fifty, I felt and looked great. I ate healthily, exercised regularly, had thick, shiny hair and great skin, and was energetic. I was working a full-time job, raising my daughter as a single mother, volunteering for the PTA, and maintaining a robust social life. My periods were regular, other than the usual PMS symptoms like cramps and bloating. I had no health complaints.

Then, I turned fifty, and things changed overnight. Literally. Overnight. I started to struggle with brain fog and low energy. I started tossing and turning for hours at night. I would wake in the middle of the night drenched in sweat! After eight or more hours in bed, I didn't feel like I was getting quality sleep and was exhausted. My moods would swing from outrage that there were no ripe avocados at Whole Foods to crying over my favorite jeans not fitting. I started to notice wrinkles and dullness in my skin, and along with that, acne—are you kidding me? My breasts grew two cup sizes, and I started having autoimmune gut issues.

After a couple of years, I found myself in the emergency room with heart palpitations. Since heart issues run in my family, I was immediately admitted. Because of my diet and lifestyle, I could not even believe I was having heart problems. After several days in the hospital, tons of blood work, EKGs, an angiogram, and a nuclear cardiac stress test that showed I have the heart of an athlete, a female cardiologist finally suggested my symptoms could be due to perimenopause. What?! I had *no idea*. I had probably been having perimenopause symptoms for years but never knew. I began to wonder: If I was struggling through midlife with all that I knew—what do other women do?

Julie

I was raised by a single mother who started her first business when she was thirty and a grandmother who earned her degree in philosophy and supported her two younger sisters through college. So I grew up being an enthusiastic advocate for women. At the University of Michigan, I tutored women who were incarcerated and teen girls who had survived abuse, and I was also a founding member of a task force that worked toward eliminating sexual assault on campus.

After college, I moved to New York City and began a career in finance. It was intense, and I was the only woman in the office. Living on pure adrenaline, I often had chest pain and felt like I was having a heart attack. But I was well compensated for the grinding work, so I explored my other passions: healing arts, quantum physics, the nature of consciousness, Tai Chi, Ayurveda, macrobiotic cooking, and more. Then I attended a weekend meditation retreat that changed my life. I began practicing meditation daily, attended a two-week silent retreat, and became a vegetarian after being a lifelong cheeseburger lover.

One evening after work, I visited my favorite bookstore and felt drawn to a beautiful book. On the cover, two hands were enveloped by light. *Hands of Light* by former NASA physicist Barbara Brennan was a life-altering book for me. I enrolled in her four-year program to study healing science. I was mentored by one of her top graduates and built a successful healing practice for many years. The majority of my clients were female, suffering from autoimmune issues, infertility, and hormonal challenges. Longing to better care for them, I studied early childhood development and trauma at the Center for Intentional Living.

When I was thirty-eight, my son was born, and my health did a wild flip. I was diagnosed with multiple issues, including an autoimmune disease. As a passionate researcher longing to regain my health, I spoke with many top physicians, read many books, and learned everything I could about postpartum, the endocrine system, hormones, the thyroid, adrenals, toxins, and digestive challenges. It was quite a perimenopausal adventure! Finally, a dear friend connected me with an excellent MD, PhD, whose practice focused on hormonal balance, environmental medicine, and longevity. Following her guidance, my health began to recover, and in six months, I felt and looked vibrant. She became my mentor, sharing with me her incredible wisdom regarding women's health and wellness.

For over thirty years, I have supported and educated women, building a team of outstanding physicians, health and life coaches, and practitioners dedicated to restoring women's health, especially during midlife. But . . . I was unprepared for the impending menopausal wave. That story comes later in the book!

Julie and Pam

We have accumulated decades of wisdom and stories to share. But during our research, neither of us found a great book co-written by two friends. Who doesn't want to learn all the juicy details from a girlfriend who has been there and done that? We thought it was time for women to get some intel on what no one tells you in midlife.

You know how during sex ed, the nurse handed out the pink book, told the girls about pads and tampons, and explained a few of your body parts? We learned about how babies are made and where they come from. Cringey as it was, at least you had an idea of what was about to happen. (Or maybe you didn't.) We had also both read books like *Our Bodies, Ourselves* and *Are You There God? It's Me, Margaret*, to help make sense of puberty and menstruation.

There are countless books available about pregnancy. There are also books on child rearing, skin care, diet, and self-help. But we asked each other: Where are the books on what to expect when you reach midlife? Where were the books about the hot flashes, body changes, anxiety, grief, and emotional roller coaster that may be worse with menopause? And what about sex and our often shifting love relationships? How about some practical info on diet and self-care for midlife women? We wanted the real details, details that addressed what we wished we had known.

Before writing this book, we interviewed hundreds of women and learned that they also wanted to know what to expect when they *weren't* expecting. We learned women wanted to know what was going on when, why and how. We learned women wanted to know the real deal on hormones and what foods to eat as their bodies were changing. Women asked about their sexuality and caring for themselves as they aged. Women told us stories of grief and longing for community and meaningful relationships. Women also wanted to know what to do in their next stage of life.

We are going to cover all of these topics, giving you the information most asked for and inspiring stories that we hope will provide insight and a sense of relatability. We have also included a QR code that will take you to our robust book portal, which is chock-full of resources, meditations, recipes, and more to help you on your journey.

Our intention for writing *Midlife Upgrade* was to share the gifts of women's combined experiences and lessons learned. We both had dramatic midlife transformations and are here to say that midlife isn't the end! It's an opportunity to transform physically, emotionally, and spiritually. If you're reaching midlife, it's time to unveil your desires and longings. Your life experience is gold, and now is the time!

Until we figure out how to extend our lifespans, midlife is when the realization of our mortality arrives. Maybe you have already been feeling nudges indicating that you are meant for more or that you want to leave a legacy behind. Fantastic! We are here to light your path. You deserve to have more love for yourself, more vibrant health, and to follow your heart's desires. Because honey, it ain't over 'til it's over.

Are you ready for an upgrade? We are ready for you!

CHAPTER 1

PERI-WHAT?

Reviewed by Vesna Skul, MD, FACP

*"Midlife is not the time to disenchant ourselves.
It's time to turn on all our magic in full force."*
—Marianne Williamson

"I was totally prepared for midlife and menopause!"
—Said by literally no woman ever

Seen in a menopause Facebook group:

- "I have been having my period for like three weeks now! WTH is going on?"
- "I was literally up all night with hot flashes and night sweats. I'm only 39, aren't I too young for this?"
- "Out of the blue, I have started getting acne everywhere—including my back and chest. Is this related to my hormones?"
- "I gained 30 pounds over the last 6 months with NO change to my diet or exercise. I'm so angry."
- "My anxiety is through the roof! I was in the ER with chest pains and the tests were all good so they sent me home, but I still feel very worried."

- "I'm 41 and have two periods each month. My doctor told me to make sure I use good birth control because my chances of getting pregnant are high right now. What the heck? I think that's bad advice."

- "At 47 I feel the worst I have felt in my life. I have constant aches and pains, headaches, bloating, and cramping. I'm not sleeping and I have zero libido. My doctor told me to take naps and Advil. I'm trying to hold down a full-time job and I am losing my shit over here."

- "Why are my 40s so hard? I sat at my desk and burst into tears. I just feel like I'm letting everyone down and I'm so tired and frustrated."

- "I am wondering—how in the hell did our moms deal with this shit? I don't remember her saying anything—did that generation just grin and bear it? Because this sucks."

- "Sleep? What is sleep? Asking for a friend."

Well, at least one woman had a sense of humor.

Pam

If I really think back on it, my perimenopause probably started in my early forties. I first noticed a pretty big drop in my energy. I always had enormous amounts of energy and did not require much sleep. Granted, I was doing a lot at the time—working, raising my daughter, volunteering, making time to spend with friends, and getting up at 5:00 a.m. for early morning exercise classes—so I chalked up the low energy to just doing too much. When I mentioned it to my friends, they said they were feeling the same way and simply reminded me we are all getting older, so I dismissed it as a symptom of aging.

The next shift I remember noticing was intense brain fog and forgetfulness. I would forget what I was saying mid-sentence, and my mind would go completely blank. I would be in the middle of a sales presentation and completely lose my train of thought. Or I would walk into a room and have no idea why I went in there. I had always had a fantastic memory, and suddenly it felt like my brain had gone offline. I wondered if I had the beginning stages of dementia or Alzheimer's. Seriously—it was that bad!

I chalked up my energy and brain issues to diet and lifestyle. Even though I was a relatively healthy person, I started looking for things I could do to get healthier because I was not about to let aging slow me down! I tidied up my diet, amped up the exercise, and barely consumed alcohol or sweets. And do you want to know what happened? By my late forties, I had gained twenty pounds and my breasts had grown by two cup sizes! It was all fun and games until my gorgeous lingerie from France didn't fit anymore.

They say hindsight is twenty-twenty. Now I know I was *definitely* in perimenopause; I just didn't know it then. And I'm not alone.

Us

In 2021, AARP[1] surveyed women over thirty-five and found that only 18% said they felt "very informed" about the impact of hormones on aging, which means a whopping 82% have no idea what is about to happen (or what is already happening)! 58% of the women interviewed said they wanted more information about the physical aspects of hormonal changes and an even larger percentage, 61%, wanted information on how hormones impact mental health. You can bet your bottom dollar your hormones affect your brain.

The initial menopause symptoms, known as perimenopause, can start eight to twelve years before actual menopause starts, and 85% of women experience symptoms during the transition. By the way, the average length of perimenopause is seven and a half years, so knowing your body and what is happening during this time can help relieve some of the anxiety around the abrupt and slow-onset changes.[2] Many women are completely caught off guard because they believe menopause is simply an on-off switch, but in reality, it can be a long transition.

Your hormone levels start changing earlier than you think. What?! Since no one educated us about perimenopause, we don't expect to have any symptoms until menopause hits. That is so wrong! Stay tuned for details.

Webster's Dictionary defines perimenopause as "the period around the onset of menopause that is often marked by various physical signs (such as hot flashes and menstrual irregularity)." Oh, is that all? The Oxford English Dictionary says, "The earliest known use of the noun perimenopause is in the 1960s. OED's earliest evidence for perimenopause is from 1962, in the writing of J. K. Frost." So, we can assume before the 1960s, women didn't experience perimenopause? (Cue laughter.)

According to the National Institutes of Health, the number of women in menopause is huge. Fifty million women are currently navigating menopause, and every year, another 2.2 million join the ranks. And this is just in the United States. The United Nations estimates there are currently over one billion (!) women internationally experiencing menopause.[3] While not every woman will experience childbirth, 100% of women with ovaries will experience menopause, and yet somehow it has remained a taboo subject.

According to the Bonafide 2021 study, "The State of Menopause," relatively few women are even talking about this subject.[4] This study found that 29% of women never sought out information on menopause, almost half (45%) didn't know the difference between perimenopause and menopause, 20% experienced symptoms before being evaluated by a health care provider, and 34% had never been diagnosed as menopausal. The majority, a whopping 73% (!), said they weren't treating any of their symptoms. That is a hell of a lot of women suffering! Menopause can be such a big transition in a woman's life, so it's about time to start giving it the attention it deserves.

Let's get clear here—perimenopause is a natural process leading up to menopause, which marks the end of your menstrual cycle. This transitional process is when your ovaries stop releasing eggs in preparation for shutting down. During perimenopause, you may begin to feel, well, let's just say it like it is—crappy. It's the change before the change or the real hell before the moderate hell of menopause. It's the surprise party you didn't ask for and don't want to attend. You are just minding your own business, and suddenly your body decides it's going to throw a hormonal jamboree. Only there are no streamers or cake. And you are *not* having a good time. Remember how during puberty, you were like, "What the hell is going on?" Well, it's a little like that. In reverse.

Before we go further, we want to give you a primer on female hormones so you can begin to make sense of what is happening. We are going to dive much deeper into hormones later, but here are some basics. The three primary female reproductive hormones are estrogen, progesterone, and testosterone. In women, these are mainly produced in the ovaries and are responsible for a host of operations: puberty, pregnancy, sex drive, hair growth, bone and muscle growth, body fat distribution, inflammatory response, cholesterol levels, and, yes, even menopause. Your hormones do a lot in your body! Since perimenopause is the time when your ovaries are shutting down, you can see why you might be feeling lousy.

Perimenopause is a completely normal process despite what it may feel like. But you should be aware of what is going on so that you aren't completely shocked when your body starts changing. The reality is that while most women know what menopause is, they just don't know what to expect or when to expect it. The best thing you can do is educate yourself and implement healthy lifestyle choices so you can feel as good and balanced as possible before your transition even starts.

The perimenopause transition can and does vary wildly from woman to woman. Since there is no predictability whatsoever and no one really talks about it, perimenopause tends to be a baffling time for many women. Most women walk around blissfully happy until they feel like complete garbage. We recommend talking to your mother, aunt, sister, or any other female relative for some guidance since the menopause transition may be genetic.

During this wacky time, you might still be having regular periods—or not. You might experience changes in your flow, or your PMS symptoms might worsen. This is because as your ovaries are slowly shutting down, wild hormone fluctuations can contribute to a host of random symptoms.

While it's accurate that perimenopause is the time before the onset of menopause, it has been our experience that there are quite a few more signs of it than just hot flashes and menstrual irregularity. In fact, you may feel a wide variety of mood swings, from feeling emotional and weepy to irritable and anxious. For no obvious reason. There are two stages of perimenopause: early perimenopause, when your periods may still be fairly regular, and late perimenopause, when your periods may become irregular and heavier or lighter. If you are one of the rare ones who feels normal and like nothing is going on, good for you! You are part of the 5% who get off lucky. The majority of women will experience at least a few symptoms during this time. 80% of women experience a smorgasbord of random symptoms, and 5% of women will have incapacitating symptoms.[5] Sorry to be the bearers of bad news, ladies.

The symptoms may be subtle at first. Maybe you don't have as much energy as you used to; you forget what you were going to say in the middle of a sentence; you toss and turn a little more at night. Okay, not so bad. Then, there is no denying something is going on—your brain is not working; you have heart palpitations; you constantly feel anxious—and the next thing you know, you are raging because they are out of your favorite creamer at the store. We know; we have been there.

Here are some of the most common symptoms of perimenopause:

- Weight gain and/or bloating
- Digestive problems
- Hair loss
- Brittle nails
- Periods getting heavier and longer
- Periods getting lighter and shorter
- Irregular periods
- Worsening PMS (sore breasts, emotional outbursts)
- Anxiety and mood swings

- Hot flashes and night sweats
- Brain fog
- Short-term memory loss
- Difficulty concentrating
- Headaches and/or migraines
- Urinary urgency or incontinence
- Urinary Tract Infections
- Low libido
- Pelvic floor issues
- Vaginal dryness and painful sex
- Racing heart or palpitations
- Difficulty sleeping
- Acne
- Dry and itchy skin
- Body odor
- Breast pain
- Joint pain
- Loss of bone density
- Increased allergies
- Frozen shoulder
- Irritability—or as we like to call it, general bitchiness for no apparent reason

Oh—and there's even more than what's listed here. Seriously, it's no wonder women think they are going crazy during this time. Hormones can wreak havoc on your body and your brain. For some women, symptoms start as early as in their mid to late thirties. They slowly sneak up on you until feeling like crap just seems like your new normal. And no one tells you all of these issues may be related to perimenopause! Some doctors may deny it. A new study from the vaginal health company Kindra finds one in three women between the ages of forty-five and fifty-four are given an incorrect diagnosis for their symptoms.[6] Common perimenopause symptoms can be misdiagnosed as stress, depression, or anxiety—and it could be any of those as well.

We have worked with clients who were advised to take sleeping pills, antidepressants, and/or birth control, try yoga, or "manage their stress better" when sharing symptoms with their doctors. It's not unusual for women to spend several years and go through multiple doctors just trying to get a diagnosis or relief from their symptoms. While tests aren't necessarily critical to diagnose perimenopause, your doctor might order bloodwork to see where your hormone levels are.

In 2019, the Mayo Clinic published a paper called "Barriers to the Care of Menopausal Women," which you can find on the National Institutes of Health website.[7] It pretty much sums up why women aren't getting the care they need (and deserve). First of all, the study acknowledges that physicians tend to treat the patient and not their symptoms. The study reviews twenty residency programs in the United States and finds that while most residents agreed upon the importance of training in menopausal management, there were important knowledge gaps and a need for improvement. A study by Johns Hopkins showed that fewer than one in five doctors receive any training on perimenopause or menopause.[8] Another big problem with management is that no particular medical specialty owns the perimenopause/menopause space. What's a woman to do?

So, not only are you not informed, but you also don't really get any warning. And if you are informed and you do ask the right questions, you might still be dismissed or denied treatment. Unfortunately, in the medical world, there is a long history of women being ignored or dismissed. It's an even bigger issue for women of color, Latina women, and heavier women. That's why it's so important to educate yourself—so you can be your advocate. Hey, we deserve to have our voices heard and receive proper treatment. Quality of life is essential!

Lifestyle changes are strongly recommended during this transition. As your ovaries decrease in optimal function and your estrogen drops, your risk for high blood pressure, high cholesterol, and osteoporosis goes up. Studies show that women with healthier lifestyles generally experience lower stress levels, have fewer symptoms, and are better able to navigate the ones they do have, which is why we cover nutrition and self-care in this book.

We will cover the major symptoms of perimenopause here. We strongly encourage you to keep a list of any symptoms you are experiencing and, for heaven's sake, talk to a doctor who is educated on menopause. Some symptoms can be indications of something serious, so now is not the time to suck it up and push through.

Hot Flashes

The number one symptom (and the one that gets the most attention) of perimenopausal women is hot flashes, and according to Johns Hopkins University, they affect up to 75% of women.[9] Hot flashes are correlated to changing levels of estrogen, and they can be fairly mild or so severe that they result in sleeplessness and immediate sweating. Hot flashes can come with increased heart rate or palpitations, skin crawling, anxiety, and even nausea. And the crazy thing is, when they pass, you may feel a chill. They tend to become more frequent as you approach menopause, and for some women, they may go away a year or two after menopause. They can be brought on by stress or anxiety (other perimenopause symptoms), adrenal stress, high sugar intake, spicy foods, alcohol, tightly fitting clothes, hot weather, and caffeine. Smokers also have higher incidences of hot flashes, which, incidentally, may or may not be related to disrupted hormone levels.

We have both experienced hot flashes, and we wish we had a magical remedy for you! Some supplements may help; however, we advise you to use any supplement with caution and always speak with your doctor. Some simple things that worked for us were taking deep breaths, opening a window, taking off a layer of clothing (when possible), and splashing some cool water on our faces.

Amy's Story

After weeks of waking up soaking wet with a pounding headache and unable to muster the energy or the emotional stamina to get through my day, I knew something had to change. I did what I always do when it comes to female-related stuff—I called my girlfriends. "Are you having hot flashes?" "Are you PMSing to the nth degree?" "Are you able to sleep at night?" "What are you doing about it?" The responses were all over the board, but it was clear there was no one answer and no quick fix to this issue.

So then I started to call my health professionals. I went to my traditional Western gynecologist, and he told me that because I have a family history of breast cancer, I am not a candidate for hormone replacement. He offered me the birth control pill as a form of hormones instead, which didn't make sense to me, so I politely declined it.

I went to my integrative doctor, and she gave me some supplements to try, but they didn't touch my symptoms.

In a desperate quest for relief, a friend recommended antidepressants, which did alleviate my hot flashes but left me feeling emotionally muted and with diminished libido. Unwilling to accept this compromised state as my new normal, I embarked on a personal research journey, determined to unravel the mysteries of menopause.

I am a health and wellness professional and have been an active participant in my own health and well-being my entire life. I learned to meditate at eighteen years old and to practice yoga at twenty-three, eventually teaching both in addition to becoming a birth doula. As someone deeply committed to my well-being as well as that of others, I was surprised by the scarcity of information and the conflicting opinions on perimenopause and menopause among doctors. Determined to feel better and not accept the status quo, I continued to talk with other women, gather my data through personal research, and seek out highly recommended medical professionals.

Eight years, four doctors, and numerous trial-and-error attempts later, I finally found the right blend of hormone replacement therapy tailored to my unique needs. It became clear that listening to my body and discerning what worked best were my most reliable guides.

The point of my story is *don't give up*. This is a newer field, and there is no right answer or singular protocol. Every person and body is different, so you have to find what works for you, and it's a process. But you can feel better, and you will feel better—and I promise it's worth it.

—Amy Owen, yoga instructor and birth coach

Sleep Disturbances

Let's not forget about another super common perimenopause symptom: sleep disturbances. You crawl into bed, exhausted from a long day. You fluff your pillow and settle in for dreamland . . . only to find yourself wide awake. You toss and turn like a rotisserie chicken, trying to find the "perfect" position where you will fall asleep—but it doesn't exist. Thank you to the brain chatters, anxiety, hot flashes, and night sweats. Oh, and the urge to get up and pee. Sleepless nights are so frustrating, and lack of sleep is one of the culprits behind midlife weight gain.

If you are experiencing night after night of restless sleep, you guessed it: you might be in perimenopause. Honey, you deserve to get some sleep. It's important for cognition, mood, mental health, and cellular repair. We are going to dive much deeper into sleep in Chapter Five, which is all about self-care—so stay tuned!

Mood Changes

And then there are the mood swings that seemingly come out of nowhere. One minute, you feel like laughing hysterically, and the next minute, you're crying over a Hallmark commercial. Or, one minute, you're dancing around to your favorite song, and then you're raging in the grocery store parking lot because someone just took your space. Steadily decreasing progesterone and sporadically fluctuating estrogen and testosterone levels may be the culprit. Hormones play a bigger role than you think in the neurotransmitters in the brain. Just like when you were a moody teenager, you may be a moody menopausal woman!

Because perimenopause is already a stressful time, you might overlook how this affects your mental health. Some mood swings are normal. However, the incidence of depression goes up during perimenopause, even in women who have not experienced it before. Women who suffer postpartum depression might be more sensitive to hormone fluctuations and, therefore, can be at a higher risk for experiencing anxiety or depression during this time.[10]

Depression can manifest as a loss of interest in activities you usually enjoy, an inability to get up and go about your day, over or undereating, sleeping more than usual, an inability to fall and stay asleep, and an unusual lack of energy. When you notice a shift in your mental well-being, we urge you to seek help from a medical professional if things progress. During this time, menopause can be misdiagnosed as depression, and depression can also be misdiagnosed as menopause. But if the symptoms are prevalent and persistent, don't just shrug it off as a symptom of menopause—it's important to treat your mental health alongside your physical health.

Irregular Periods

Another thing no one tells you about is irregular periods. Believe it or not, this is also one of the hallmark signs of perimenopause. Because your estrogen levels are fluctuating wildly, this messes with the rhythm of your menstrual cycle. So, you can have skipped periods, super heavy

periods, super light periods, spotting between periods, and periods that last longer—or shorter.

In her NYT best-selling book, *How to Menopause*, Tamsen Fadal tells her story about having irregular periods. "I used to be able to time my cycle to the day. I would feel some cramps, and within an hour, my period would come. In three or four days it would be over, and that was how it went. Until my period took on a mind of its own. When I entered perimenopause, I bled so massively that I blew through super maxi pads and tampons."[11]

We have heard stories like this over and over. Can anyone relate?

Weight Fluctuations

During this time, you may also discover your clothes don't fit like they used to because your body has decided to go on a little adventure. The dreaded midlife weight gain. It's enough to make you consider investing in a wardrobe of stretchy pants. The struggle is real for many women, and studies show a woman can gain one to one and a half pounds per year in midlife, with the average total weight gain being between five to eight pounds.[12]

Pam

As I mentioned earlier, I gained twenty pounds pretty much out of the blue despite a healthy diet and regular exercise. The weight came on quickly but didn't seem to drop as easily as it used to. Fortunately, I was able to get my hormones back on track (more on that later), and my weight came down a bit. While it's unlikely I'll fit into my college jeans again, I'm making peace with the fact my body shape is curvier than it used to be.

Us

Some weight gain may be related to lack of sleep and, believe it or not, some of that is connected to . . . hot flashes. And you know where that weight goes? Well, it tends to go in the tummy area. The reason is that hot flashes raise your cortisol levels, which slows down your metabolism. This may also be an issue with your thyroid gland. We will discuss this further in a later chapter.

Managing diet and getting plenty of exercise is especially important during this time. We dive in deeper on those, too. Don't worry—you weathered puberty and acne, and you can get through this, too! We got you covered.

Hair Loss/Gain

Here's something super fun that you may experience: less hair on your head, but errant hairs on your chin (or chest, lips, or arms). Your body is dropping in progesterone, and estrogen is fluctuating, which affects hair growth and shedding. Interestingly, progesterone affects shedding even more than estrogen does. At the same time that progesterone is dropping and estrogen is fluctuating, you are still circulating androgen (male) hormones like testosterone, which can lead to errant chin hairs and even thinning hair. These same hormones can also affect the appearance of your hair color, texture, and even your skin. However, these conditions can also be caused by a thyroid imbalance or an autoimmune condition, so if this is happening to you, it's important to take note of this symptom.

Brain Fog

The last major symptoms we hear about are forgetfulness and brain fog. You know that feeling when you walk into a room and have no idea why you went in there? Or you forget what you were saying mid-sentence. You can't find your car keys (they are in your purse; you just put them there), you can't find your car in the parking lot (it's in the same space you always park in), or you're at the grocery store and have no idea what you went there for. ARGH! This too, my dears, will pass. For most women, once in full-blown menopause, your brain will come back. In the meantime, make sure you keep plenty of lists or use your notes app!

Here's the good news—not every woman suffers from these symptoms! In fact, more than 15% of you may get off scot-free![13] We like to call these women lucky bitches. While every woman's experience is different, most women will find their symptoms come and go. Unfortunately, there is no *definitive* test for perimenopause (yet!), and some of these symptoms may mimic thyroid problems, so it's important to test your hormones and thyroid function if you aren't feeling like your normal self. We will discuss thyroid and hormone testing in more detail in later chapters. If you are in your forties and your cycles have become irregular, varying seven or more days from your normal cycle, or you are skipping periods, you may be in perimenopause.

If you are experiencing multiple symptoms of perimenopause, you might consider making an appointment separate from your annual exam or physical. The reality is that most doctors only get fifteen to twenty minutes per patient, and they may not have the time to fully address your symptoms. Hot flashes, heart palpitations, and loss of sleep, just to name a few, can be harbingers of other long-term issues to come—so make sure you address them! There is no medal for suffering in silence. Remember, you are the expert on yourself, so speak up. And we are giving you permission right here, right now, to fire your doctor if they don't help you or are dismissive.

It is so important to track your symptoms during this transition so you can share any issues you're having with your healthcare provider. Fortunately, there are more and more doctors going into this field who are willing to listen, make helpful suggestions, and help relieve you of your annoying symptoms. You are entitled to live a happy, productive life, and there is no good reason to suffer when solutions are available.

Here is a perimenopause symptom tracker you might find useful. Click on the QR code at the end of the book to download a PDF of this symptoms list.

PERIMENOPAUSE SYMPTOM TRACKING LIST

SYMPTOM	FRE-QUENTLY	OFTEN	SOME-TIMES	RARELY	NEVER
Hot flashes					
Night sweats					
Heart palpitations					
Difficulty sleeping					
Fatigue					
Anxiety or panic					
Brain fog/difficulty concentrating					
Low libido					
Period changes					
Weight gain					
UTIs					
Urinary urgency					
Breast pain/tenderness					
Irritability					
Feel unhappy/depressed					
Dizzy/faint					
Muscle/joint pain					
Memory loss					
Acne					
Vaginal dryness					
Changes in skin					
Changes in hair					
Tinnitus					
Headaches					
Increased body odor					

Perimenopause pro tip: If you don't want to get pregnant, still use birth control, because yes, you can still get pregnant during this time! Pam had a friend in her late thirties who had a three-year-old brother. Her mom had thought she was too old to get pregnant at fifty—even though she still had periods—and surprise!

Here's the deal. Know that you are not alone. Just simply having some knowledge about what is going on might help you feel better. While we have discussed the physical and mental symptoms of perimenopause, other powerful changes are happening, too! Stay tuned.

CHAPTER 2

ENDOCRINE HARMONY

Reviewed by Vesna Skul, MD, FACP

"When women take care of their health, they become their own best friend."
—Maya Angelou

Both of us have learned that a woman's challenges with her hormonal journey may begin even before her first period ("menarche") and then may continue with pregnancy, birth, postpartum, perimenopause, and ... menopause. All of these stages impact our bodies physiologically. We have also discovered that to have a healthier and happier menopause, it is essential to educate ourselves about various endocrine glands: pituitary, thyroid, adrenals, and ovaries. When these glands are functioning well, our endocrine system is better equipped to smoothly hum along during perimenopause and menopause. If there are imbalances or dysfunctions with these glands, then there may be health issues during the menopausal years.

We are lucky to have been in the health space for years, and the endocrine system has always been a big topic of conversation. However, when speaking with clients, we have learned that most women have very little knowledge about it and what it does. For starters, our amazing endocrine system is made up of a network of glands and organs that produce, store, and secrete important hormones that regulate the functions of our bodies, such as metabolism, growth, sleep, reproduction, and stress response; therefore, any imbalance will impact our menopausal experience. Our endocrine system changes as we age, and we feel it is essential to give you a primer so that you can be more empowered to make informed health choices during your menopausal years.

Fair warning here: This chapter may be a bit overwhelming. We are going to share a lot of information with you, which may seem a bit dense but will be enlightening—because you should know and understand your own body. We hope that this will help you ask better questions of your practitioners and take much better care of yourself.

Julie

During my early perimenopausal journey, like so many women, I lived it! I experienced complications during the birth of my son, postpartum challenges, autoimmune thyroid issues, imbalances with my hormonal system, adrenal fatigue, and other health concerns that were undiagnosed or incorrectly treated. More importantly, I learned to be a fierce advocate for myself, dedicated to untangling and healing my challenges, and for 12 years of my late perimenopause and early menopause, I was super healthy.

During my pregnancy, my OB/GYN told me I had a somewhat low-functioning thyroid gland. He didn't seem very concerned but did share some frightening info that this might cause a miscarriage. It was over 20 years ago, and looking back, I could have pushed him for more guidance. Fortunately, I experienced a healthy, happy pregnancy and had a twenty-six-hour-long but very gentle labor—until the finale. After giving birth to my son, my placenta would not release. Years later, I discovered it might have been due to my age (thirty-eight) and the very long labor. Little did I know, I was most likely in perimenopause. No comment on the term "geriatric pregnancy."

Subsequently, I had two postpartum hemorrhages. The bleeding just wouldn't stop. I spiked a high fever, and even though I was in love with my baby boy, my body was beginning to crash, deflating from the former joy of pregnancy. I left the hospital thirty-six hours later and began motherhood. Luckily, I had my mother, sister, and husband supporting me, but my recovery took years into perimenopause.

Unbelievably, approximately 18% of births involve postpartum hemorrhages.[14] And in the immediate postpartum period, 87-94% of women report at least one health problem.[15] Long-term health problems (persisting after six months postpartum) are reported by 31% of women.[16] For nine years after my son's birth, I struggled with many debilitating health challenges. I lost most of the hair on the top of my head. I briefly went on antidepressants and was ultimately diagnosed with an autoimmune condition that had affected my thyroid, which adversely affected my entire body. My primary function was taking care of my dear son. The truth was, I couldn't do much else.

And the bottom line is that some of the health challenges I experienced can affect women whether they have given birth or not. For any new mother, caring for a newborn is challenging, especially if she has had a difficult delivery. But a difficult delivery coupled with an autoimmune illness, likely during perimenopause, almost put me over the edge.

While doing my research, I discovered a book called *Molecules of Emotion* written by Candace Pert in 1997. It was a pioneering work and, at the time, far beyond anything that had ever been written about the mind-body connection. It included comprehensive information about the hypothalamic, pituitary, and adrenal (HPA) axis as well as a description of the endocrine system, which fascinated me.[17] Unfortunately, Pert was outcast by the National Institutes of Health, as many great thinkers are when they're on the fringes of accepted "truth."

Additionally, I read *Depression After Childbirth* by Katharina Dalton, whose premise was that postpartum depression is a hormonal imbalance.[18] She, too, did a deep dive into the HPA axis and the entire endocrine system. As part of my health journey, I also interviewed authors of bestselling books and vigilantly searched for answers. I believed I would not even live another ten years, and my deepest longing was to live long enough to enjoy my future grandchildren.

Holding that intention in my heart, I finally cracked the code! Balancing my pituitary, thyroid, adrenals, and hormones, plus taking some pretty cool, cutting-edge supplements, thankfully, has paved the way for a happier menopause. Having done my research to care for myself, I understood the hormonal systems in my body that had gone offline. I advocated for myself and found some amazing, badass female doctors who listened to me, and I was therefore more equipped for the coming menopausal changes. Many of us are completely in the dark about these systems before menopause even begins. So let's dive in.

Us

Many of us are living longer lives and are committed to maintaining our health as we age. Let's get into some juicy information that will offer a deeper understanding of the changes that are going on with our bodies. Consider it your health class for midlife but without the annoying giggles, coughs, and funny looks from the boys!

It wasn't until 1993 that a federal mandate required researchers to include women and minorities in clinical research. In 2014, the National Institutes of Health *finally* created a gynecological branch to look at the health of the vulva, vagina, ovaries, and uterus. Before 2014, medical research on women's health had been focused mainly on fertility and pregnancy. As Rachel E. Gross elucidates in *Vagina Obscura*, "As a result, there are parts of your own body less known than the bottom of the ocean, or the surface of Mars."[19]

Do you even know what your uterus looks like? This beautiful illustration shows what a marvel of design and function the female anatomy truly is. It's something to be celebrated. The uterus is a muscular organ that can expand and contract as needed through the cycles of fertility and pregnancy. The female anatomy exhibits remarkable resilience and adaptability with its rhythm and renewal through each cycle from menarche to menopause. It's one of nature's most elegant designs.

FEMALE ANATOMY OF THE UTERUS

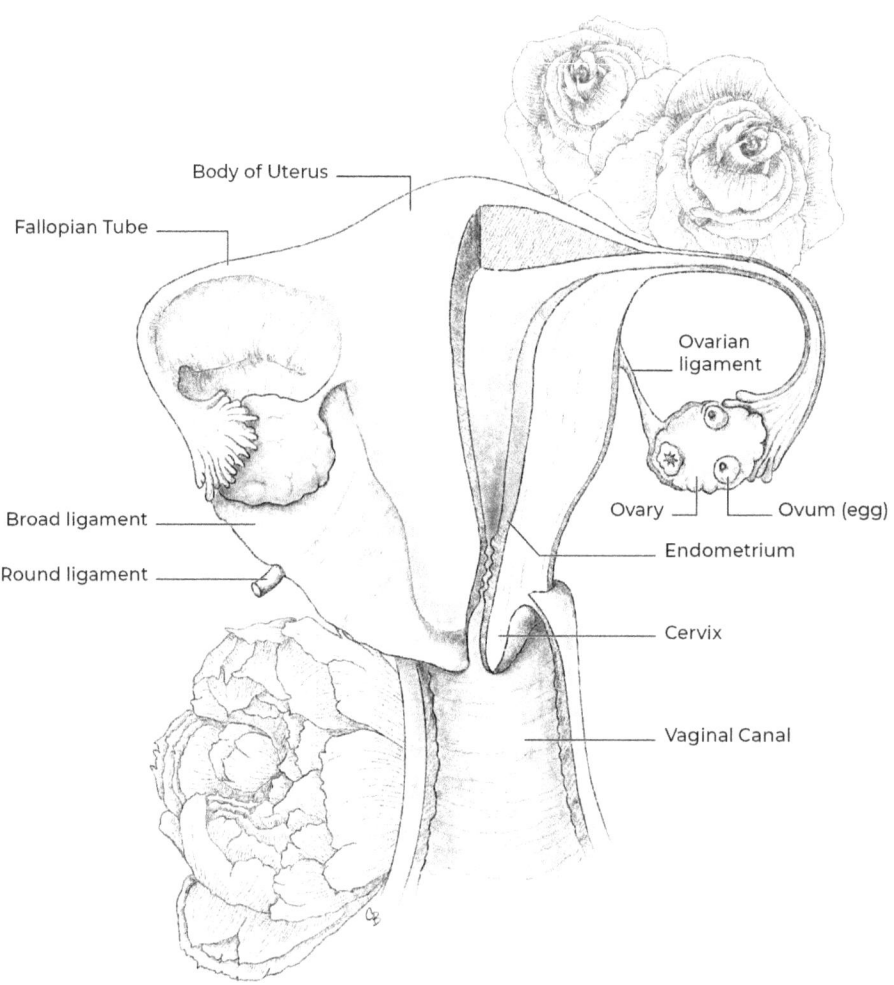

"The broad ligament is one of my favorite ligaments within the human body. It almost seems as if the broad ligament is giving a hug to the uterus. As the broad ligament hugs the uterus, it provides essential vascular support to the ovaries, uterus, and fallopian tubes while physically holding these structures together."

—Clara Baumgarten, MS

We are pretty sure your health class also did not include a download on your endocrine system, and we bet you didn't learn about menopause, either. So now we are going to unpack the endocrine system, reviewing the pituitary, thyroid, adrenals, and ovaries, their connection with each other, and how they affect your health during midlife. Consider it sex education 101 for your anatomy!

FEMALE ENDOCRINE SYSTEM

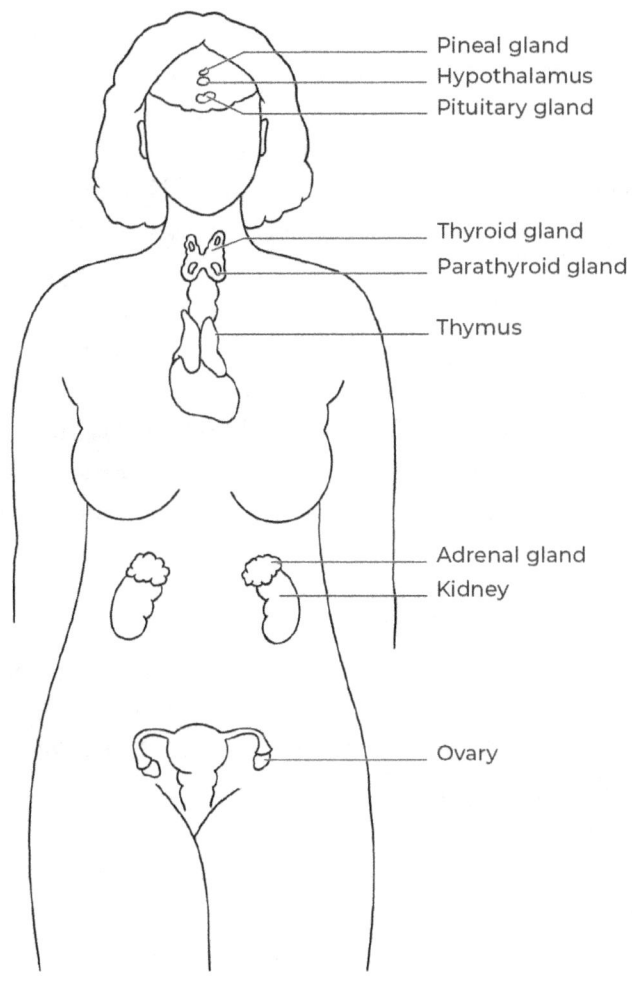

Julie

PITUITARY GLAND

If I had to pick a favorite endocrine gland, it would have to be the glorious pituitary. I fell in love with the pituitary and its friend, the pineal gland, when I was studying in the late '80s with NASA physicist and author of two bestsellers, Barbara Brennan. She wrote *Hands of Light* and *Light Emerging*, and she quantified the human energy field, including what we now know as the ancient Vedic chakra system. The word chakra means a subtle energy center, also referred to as a wheel of light, and was not yet being casually tossed around on blogs—or even yoga classes—in the late '80s. While Americans might have "discovered" chakras in the '80s, the wisdom of the chakra system is thousands of years older than the Roman Empire! While training with Barbara, I became very aware of the importance of a healthy pituitary and its correlation to subtle energies for the third eye chakra, located in the middle of the forehead.

The pituitary is about the size of a pea, located at the base of the brain and connected to the hypothalamus. Considered the master gland, some of our doctor friends have called it the "conductor of the hormonal symphony." It sits in a little bony cradle called the sella turcica and is responsible for producing several hormones. It tells the other endocrine glands (such as the thyroid, ovaries, and adrenals) to produce and release their hormones.

If the pituitary is imbalanced, that will affect our entire endocrine system. The pituitary can go offline due to stress or traumatic brain injury, and it can become damaged during a difficult birthing experience when a mother is forcibly pushing during the final stages of delivery. This increased pressure leads to a lack of blood supply to the pituitary, causing atrophy and the subsequent reduction of essential hormones necessary for our health.

The pituitary and the frontal cortex communicate through intricate microvascular connections. Not surprisingly, the third eye chakra, located in the area of the frontal cortex, is believed to support clear thinking, insight, wisdom, open-mindedness, and the ability to visualize and create a beautiful future for ourselves. If you are having issues with feeling stuck or trapped in your life, unable to access your inner wisdom, or are feeling depressed or even anxious, you might have an imbalance in this chakra. Take note because you might also have issues with your pituitary gland, as it produces several neurotransmitters (such as dopamine, acetylcholine, and GABA) responsible for mood, focus, concentration, and thought processing speed.

THYROID GLAND

I learned the hard way that it is vital to maintain the health of my thyroid after struggling for years with an autoimmune condition called Hashimoto's thyroiditis (now in total remission). Hashimoto's is an inflammation of the thyroid gland. The thyroid is shaped like a butterfly and is located at the front center of your neck. It is the thermostat that regulates the energy for your entire body. It directly controls your metabolism and indirectly controls mood, menstrual cycles, and many other essential functions of your body. There are four common thyroid problems:

- Hypothyroidism: an under-functioning of the thyroid gland
- Hashimoto's: an autoimmune form of hypothyroidism
- Hyperthyroidism: an over-functioning of the thyroid gland
- Grave's disease: an autoimmune form of hyperthyroidism

Thyroid disease affects around thirty million people in the United States, and 90% of them are women.[20] Hypothyroidism is also most common in middle-aged, perimenopausal women. Thyroid disorders can impact the risk of long-term complications of menopause, such as osteoporosis and cardiovascular disease. Having autoimmune Hashimoto's or Grave's disease also increases your risk for other autoimmune diseases and complications. Issues with hypothyroidism can lead to severe exhaustion, impacting everything in a person's life, especially during midlife. Low thyroid function affects our cognitive abilities, memory, and focus. When I had undiagnosed Hashimoto's, my brain often felt scrambled. I would think I was saying the word "dog," and I'd say "tennis" instead. Very scary.

Thyroid issues can also mess with our hormones and metabolism and prevent ovulation from occurring, therefore affecting fertility. We have supported many clients who were dismissed by their doctors when they raised their concerns about the correlation between the thyroid and infertility. As an OB/GYN shared with us, research shows that women who have thyroid issues can be more likely to have challenges getting pregnant and have a higher risk for miscarriage when the issues are untreated. We always share with our clients and friends that the thyroid is the gas pedal for the body. Many women who are hypothyroid or have Hashimoto's are more susceptible to depression and weight gain, even if they make healthy lifestyle choices.

Working with many women over the years, we found that thyroid disease is an often undiagnosed epidemic in this country. Even if you are feeling a little "off," it is *super* important that you have your thyroid function checked immediately. I waited a year, and a lot of unnecessary damage was done. Many doctors will *only* test your thyroid-stimulating hormone (TSH), but the complete thyroid panel below has been recommended to us. We hope sharing this with you now will lead you to a timely and proper diagnosis with appropriate treatment if necessary.

Many women are undiagnosed and suffer for years because their lab tests are within "normal" ranges, and again, their physicians may only test TSH. The full lab panel is necessary if you are having any of the following symptoms of Hashimoto's: hair loss, thinning eyebrows, constipation, big-time ongoing fatigue, weight gain, cold hands and feet, depression, mental sluggishness, cognitive dysfunction, slow reflexes, hoarse voice, low immunity, and menstrual irregularities, among others. And for hyperthyroidism: accelerated metabolism, weight loss, anxiety, rapid heart rate, tremors, skin changes, excess sweating, heavy periods, and bulging eyes.

A complete Thyroid Panel includes:

- TSH
- Free T3

- Reverse T3
- Free T4
- Thyroid peroxidase antibodies
- Antithyroglobulin antibodies

Dr. Aviva Romm, author of the insightful book *Adrenal Thyroid Revolution*, writes, "You are the expert of your own body. It's your doctor's JOB to listen and to give you the trust, support, information, and access to resources you need to help you live your best life. That's what the whole medical profession should be about."[21] Indeed, a shift like that does constitute a revolution. Romm also has an outstanding website with an abundance of educational blog posts.

After decades of coaching women, we have observed correlations between their thyroid disorders and their inability to use their voices. They have trouble speaking their truth, singing, laughing, vocalizing pleasure with orgasm, and, very importantly, owning their power. Our bodies do have incredible wisdom. It is no coincidence that thyroid challenges for women are epidemic. It is absolutely time to speak our truth.

Louise Hay, an innovator in the consciousness movement, wrote the amazing book *You Can Heal Your Life*. In it, she shares the following question for those with thyroid issues to contemplate: "I never get to do what I want to do. When is it my turn?" If you have thyroid issues, consider this important question. The mind-body connection is powerful.

There has been very little research on the root causes of why autoimmune issues for women are escalating globally. It is known that women are particularly vulnerable to environmental toxins as a result of exposure to pesticides, herbicides, heavy metals, bisphenol A (BPA), phthalates, and more. Many toxins, called xenoestrogens, mimic estrogen and tie up the estrogen receptor sites in the body, contributing to hormonal chaos. BPA and phthalates are both present in plastics, and there are many phthalates in our personal care products. So start reading labels, and consider getting rid of household cleaners that can be toxic and, sorry to say, your glamorous and pricey shampoos, perfumes, and skincare products that have a long list of funky ingredients. And you most definitely do not want to be using toxic pesticides in your garden!

As you optimize your thyroid function, you will be offering your body the support it needs to be healthier during your perimenopausal years and beyond. As mentioned earlier, many thyroid issues are often undiagnosed. So if you are experiencing any of the symptoms of thyroid imbalances, please contact your healthcare provider immediately. We have had many clients who had undiagnosed thyroid challenges; as they cleared up their issues, they became much healthier, and their menopausal journeys therefore became gentler.

Adrenal Glands

The adrenal glands are a pair, each located just above the kidney. They produce more than eighty substances, including hormones that regulate the immune system, stress responses, metabolism, blood sugar, and energy. During perimenopause and menopause, the adrenal glands may overwork, compensating for lower hormonal levels and undergoing additional stress. When our adrenals were taxed, both of us experienced being incredibly fatigued, but at the same time, we felt like we were hyped up on caffeine.

As women, we do so very much in all areas of our lives, and we can endure stress, stress, and more stress. For many of us, the pandemic blew out our adrenals, which could have been compromised already. You, too, may be recovering from the tsunami of cortisol, produced by the adrenals, that has rolled through your body for many years. Chronic stress has a complex effect on the body. It doesn't simply wear out the adrenals. It can interfere with our hormone production as well as impact other parts of the body.

In our early years, our adrenals were likely pumping along reasonably well. They are quite resilient and can tolerate a lot, but when enough is enough, our bodies can go into chaos and create health issues that contemporary medicine finds hard to resolve. According to the National Library of Medicine, chronic stress is a common risk factor in 75-90% of all diseases.[22]

Almost all adrenal fatigue treatments are marketed toward midlife women. Start talking with a friend about your exhaustion, and your social media algorithm will pop up with targeted ads for energy drinks, sleep gummies (some are great!), cooling pillows, and all manner of possible solutions that will not directly address your adrenal dysfunction.

Often, adrenal fatigue is not recognized as valid. Women may be given a diagnosis of Addison's disease, which reflects virtually zero adrenal function due to autoimmune destruction of the adrenals, or Cushing's syndrome, which is characterized by sky-high cortisol levels. A physician once told our client, "Your adrenals are tanked. That happens when you are exposed to long-term chronic stress." The symptoms of chronic stress are a consequence of being in a constant state of fight or flight and may manifest as anxiety, extreme fatigue, insomnia, weight gain around our waist, brain fog, jacked-up blood sugar, havoc with our hormones that may cause suppressed thyroid function, and decreased sex drive. These symptoms are also very common in perimenopause and menopause, so make sure you track your symptoms, talk to your (understanding) practitioner, and get your labs done!

Both of us had adrenals that were definitely "tanked" during perimenopause, and they are much happier and healthier now. We have taken steps to heal our adrenals by restoring proper thyroid function, optimizing our pituitary function, having great sleep hygiene, and reducing our caffeine intake. Any modalities that promote deep relaxation and restore balance to the nervous system by activating the parasympathetic arm of our autonomic nervous system—such as meditation (mindfulness, Transcendental Meditation, and others), yoga, breathwork, and somatic healing—are steps in the right direction. There are also restorative Ayurvedic and Chinese herbs that are very effective for bringing your adrenals back online. Listen to your body.

We can't say it enough. Practice self-care, dear ones. Even simple actions can make your life easier. Know that with proper self-care, good nutrition, and plenty of rest, you can restore your adrenal power during perimenopause and menopause.

Ovaries

Betty White once wrote that her mother used to say, "The older you get, the better you get. Unless you are a banana." We would add... unless you are an ovary. Keep this in mind as we go into detail about our ovaries.

Our beautiful and bountiful ovaries are mainly responsible for producing eggs and secreting sex hormones that promote fertility. Menopause occurs when the ovaries run out of eggs and then out of business! Did you know that we are born with our entire lifetime supply of eggs? In our mother's womb, each of us had our ovaries filled with six to seven million oocytes (eggs).[23] Our mothers carried not only our eggs but also the eggs of our future children. At birth, we were left with about a million, and at puberty, we had approximately 350,000.[24] Our eggs start dying off at the rate of 1000 per menstrual cycle. Approximately 400 eggs go through the process of ovulation, and between the ages of forty-five to fifty-five, the majority of us run out of eggs completely.

Since some women born today might have a potential life expectancy of 100 years or more, these women will be living over half their lives in menopause.[25] What if we could extend the life of our ovaries? It's some wild science, but this may be possible in the future. Some very compassionate scientists around the world are doing pioneering work in this field.

"For women, aging is intimately associated with the ovaries. And unlike most other tissues of the body, the ovaries age long before anything else."[26] This was a shocker for us: The ovaries age at twice the rate of the rest of the organs! Doesn't that seem like a glitch in the matrix for women and our longevity? According to advocates for women's health and longevity experts, doctors Garrison, Delucia, and La Folette, the age at which a woman goes through menopause is directly correlated with her lifespan.[27] If you go through menopause later, you will tend to live longer.

The ovaries not only produce, store, and release eggs, but they also produce hormones that impact the health of the organs in the body, from the bones to the brain. That's why menopausal women are more susceptible to osteoporosis, cardiovascular disease, dementia, and other symptoms that can contribute to menopausal hell.

Some data suggests stressors that can accelerate ovarian aging also include our food choices, environmental toxin load, disrupted sleep, and lack of exercise.[28] Gentle upgrades to our lifestyle choices can have profound effects on our well-being and will support hormonal balance and menstrual health and, therefore, healthy ovarian function. If lengthening the ovarian lifespan becomes possible, women might be able to live healthier lives and avoid some of the serious health challenges associated with menopause.

HPA Axis

The hypothalamic-pituitary-adrenal (HPA) axis sounds complicated (and it is), but we will keep it simple. Knowing the basics about how it functions will help you to be an advocate for your health during midlife. The HPA axis helps to regulate our body's response to stress by controlling the stress response. Some of the symptoms of a challenged HPA axis might include not being able to cope well with stress, deep fatigue, feeling irritable and overwhelmed by frequent illnesses, and lowered immunity. Dysfunction in the HPA axis can be one of the primary reasons for hormonal imbalance, especially during perimenopause and menopause.

Our physiological reaction to stress is a survival mechanism for the body, and this response protects us from internal and external dangers. Our neurochemical and hormonal reactions to stress have not changed much since the beginning of humanity, but what drives those reactions has. Our ancient ancestors might have been running from a dangerous animal, but today, it could be about responding to a multitude of intense acute and chronic stressors. As a woman, you may be dealing with difficult relationships, sleeping issues, work demands, blood sugar instability due to poor eating habits, the daily barrage of bad news, and all of the challenges of living in the twenty-first century. You get the picture.

The HPA axis, designed to keep our bodies in top condition for extreme and temporary stress, can be knocked out of whack due to chronic stress, triggering multiple symptoms and placing increased demands on the pituitary, adrenals, and hypothalamus. As a consequence of chronic stress, cortisol levels become elevated. Our bodies cannot tolerate acute stressors, and it takes longer for stress-induced cortisol to return to normal levels.[29] So, the adrenals are pumping out a lot of cortisol, and with this excessive exposure, metabolic and neuropsychiatric issues can develop.

In other words, long-term, chronic stress results in an over-activation of the HPA Axis and high cortisol levels, which are implicated in many different health issues. The physical experience of chronic stress will be unique to each individual. In the beginning, you may experience it as "wired but tired" followed by complete exhaustion. Your friend may experience it as intense anxiety or constant anger, and your sister may experience it as fatigue or depression.

So what does this mean for you? We believe that some of our clients in perimenopause and menopause may have HPA axis dysregulation. Dr. Aviva Romm calls this chronic sense of being overwhelmed and its downstream effects "Survival Overdrive Syndrome." Both of us have experienced the symptoms of this syndrome, and we believe that this has contributed to many of our health issues. Fortunately, we have healed and are continuing to heal ourselves by adopting strategies and suggestions we use in our program and with our coaching clients.

Postpartum

JULIE

As I mentioned, I had postpartum issues. The hemorrhages drained me. At thirty-eight, I was already struggling with little sleep and all the typical challenges of new motherhood. That's when I somehow discovered—pre-Internet and pre-Amazon—the books I mentioned earlier: *Depression After Childbirth* by Katharina Dalton and *Molecules of Emotion* by Candace Pert.

Both books toppled the paradigm that I was suffering because of some fault of my own. I learned that my postpartum struggles could be deeply rooted in hormonal imbalances. I had done everything "right" during my pregnancy, and yet, I still faced significant postpartum challenges.

Reminder: The imbalances that challenge us during menarche and the years of menses, along with fertility or infertility, pregnancy, miscarriage, childbirth, and postpartum, *may profoundly impact how we experience menopause.* To better understand our individual menopause experiences and the potential for greater health and wellness, we need to consider all of the hormonal stages that we have experienced earlier in our lives.

Unfortunate facts: The United States is the only high-income nation in the world that does not have paid maternity leave, and it is estimated that one in four women return to work within two weeks of giving birth.[30] The United States is also one of the most dangerous places to give birth, ranking behind Syria and Uzbekistan in 2020.[31] Balancing a career, managing the physical and emotional challenges of recovering from birth, and caring for a newborn all at the same time puts women at higher risk for postpartum depression (PPD).

Scientists are *now* finally acknowledging that one potential cause of postpartum depression may be fluctuating hormones and inflammation in our bodies. And just recently, in 2019, the FDA approved Brexanolone, the first drug approved for PPD, made from a derivative of the hormone progesterone.[32] It might seem like a novel breakthrough, but only two clinical trials for a small subset of women exist, no information is available for safety during breastfeeding, and the intravenous drug can cost $34,000! We most certainly have some major distance to cover and systems to dismantle for women to be cared for during postpartum and all of the stages of our lives.

Fortunately, I had a friend during my postpartum phase who was a registered nurse, Ayurvedic practitioner, and doula. She shared with me that women can have three "sacred windows" during their lifetime: menarche, pregnancy, and menopause. She believed that these times had the potential for a greater awakening to our true selves and our power as women and that if the pregnancy and postpartum were difficult and not fully resolved, we could become very depleted, and menopause could be difficult as well.

If Dr. Dalton's premise that PPD might be hormonally influenced were to be seriously considered, then women's concerns might not be so readily dismissed. We might be given better suggestions than what my endocrinologist OB/GYN recommended: "Take a long walk, and you will feel better." While PPD may be hormonally related to a sudden drop in progesterone, some women benefit from a short-term treatment of low-dose antidepressant medication (SSRIs) that could be lifesaving. More physicians are being trained to inquire about the signs and symptoms of PPD in their patients, which is finally addressing the problem and offering effective treatments.

Many other emotional factors can precipitate PPD, such as Post Traumatic Stress Disorder. As Dr. Dalton said, "We all have a responsibility to be aware of unexpected torment that can occur in a new mother's mind, leading her to act in the most unexpected way when she is at the end of her tether. More education of the public is required before there can be an end to these tragedies, which is the very reason for writing this book."[33]

Interestingly, most women have never heard of Dr. Katherina Dalton. She made huge contributions to our understanding of hormonal imbalances, coined the term PMS, and wrote *The PMS Bible*! She identified the many symptoms women may experience after childbirth as having a pattern similar to PMS. She successfully advocated for using large doses of bioidentical progesterone immediately after childbirth, especially to protect women who had a history of PMS from the precipitous drop that may occur with childbirth.

Reading Dr. Dalton's and Dr. Pert's books those years ago sparked a desire in me. I did not want any woman to suffer the way that I did. As I was breastfeeding my son, I dreamed of writing a book to support women with fertility, childbirth, and postpartum. And I couldn't write my thoughts down fast enough. This was 2001—and it would have been a hell of a lot easier with iPhone dictation, btw. Being a full-time mama and starting another business, I put that desire aside. But I carried it to this day, and now Pam and I have written this book supporting you in having a gentler midlife journey!

PAM

I had a blissful pregnancy. Seriously. People would walk up to me and tell me how beautiful and happy I looked. I loved being pregnant and everything that went with it. I enjoyed it so much that I could have lived as a pregnant woman my whole life! Unfortunately, I had a very difficult delivery. My daughter somehow flipped over before I delivered her, and she came out face up instead of face down. They had to use suction and forceps to get her out; it was very painful; and I lost a lot of blood. Gratefully, she was a very healthy, strong, and alert baby.

At first, everything was great. She nursed very easily and slept like a champ. For me, however, the bottom fell out after the first week. I was sweating like crazy every night—like through everything. I had to strip the bed every morning to wash the sweat-soaked sheets. I cried all day even though I was head over heels in love with my baby. I was despondent. I didn't know where to turn or what to do. I had the most wonderful of pregnancies—how could everything be so awful afterward? My OB/GYN wanted to put me on antidepressants, but I refused because I was nursing. So, through a lot of tears, I toughed it out, and it wasn't easy. I suffered for many months, smiling in pictures but feeling tortured inside.

Little did I know back then, my postpartum depression was most likely due to a severe drop in progesterone. Interestingly, I also suffered for years with horrible PMS, which has now also been found to be linked to low progesterone. I had the kind of PMS that would have me lying on the cold bathroom tile just for some relief. I had not the slightest inkling that my low progesterone was likely related to my postpartum depression.

Also, I have had an extremely challenging perimenopause. When I learned about the link between postpartum depression and menopause, my symptoms suddenly started to make more sense. Hormones (especially progesterone) have been a lifesaver to me in midlife. I only wish I had known about this link sooner; it might have saved me a lot of grief. I feel like every mother should know about this! It could make things so much easier for so many women. I am so grateful to have found relief with bioidentical hormones.

Us

We have spent decades learning through trial and error, because we are still living during a time that doesn't always honor the beautiful cycles of women's bodies. However, times are changing, and women are demanding more answers. We strongly encourage you to do your research, so you can be your own advocate. We have shared the experiences and knowledge that have enlightened and guided us. Our wish is that our journeys will inform yours and make it gentler.

CHAPTER 3

IT'S NOT ME. IT'S MY HORMONES!

Reviewed by Vesna Skul, MD, FACP

"Your body is breaking up with levels of hormones it has had for 30 years or longer. It's no surprise it's upset."
—Dr. Kourtney Sims

Let's get some clarity around menopause. Menopause is not the same as perimenopause. The word menopause is tossed around like it encompasses the entire menopausal experience. It does not. Perimenopause is the time leading up to menopause. And there is no such thing as post-menopause. You are qualified to be part of the menopausal club once your menses are permanently paused. Membership forever. Sorry. Yes, you are officially in menopause if you haven't had a period for twelve months. Seems a bit arbitrary to us. Why is it a year? Why isn't it six or eighteen months? And sometimes, a period will sneak back in after a year.

We have a lovely fifty-five-year-old client who was having difficult menopausal symptoms. She had been part of the menopausal club for a few years. She went for a pelvic ultrasound, and the technician couldn't find her ovaries. The tech did a deeper scan and shared that the ovaries were very small and, therefore, difficult to find. The tech shared with her—rather ungraciously, "That's what happens when you run out of eggs. Your ovaries shrivel." "Shrivel"—brush up on those communication skills, people. Menopausal women give fewer f**ks—so watch out. Okay—"shriveled" ovaries; no more eggs—and no more periods for over a year. Our dear client was definitely in menopause.

The term "menopause" wasn't coined until 1820 by a French physician, Charles de Gardanne.[34] Before then, it was colloquially referred to as "women's hell," "green old age," and "death of sex." At least in French, those references may have sounded somewhat less terrifying! Dr. Gardanne also reported fifty menopause-related conditions, including epilepsy, nymphomania, gout, and hysterical fits. We get the fits thing—but nymphomania? No comment!

The Menopause Society predicts that in 2025, over one billion women globally will be in menopause.[35] Every day in the United States, over 6,000 women, at the average age of 51, enter menopause.[36] For some of us, menopause may be the beginning of a welcome relief from perimenopausal symptoms, which may have begun over a decade earlier. For others, the challenges can continue for years. Dr. Wen Shen, gynecologist and assistant professor at the Johns Hopkins School of Medicine, says, "Nearly one-third of women in this country are menopausal. Many of them are needlessly suffering."[37] And according to an AARP study, three in four women surveyed between the ages of fifty and fifty-nine said their menopausal symptoms interfered with their lives![38]

We had perimenopausal experiences that were like walking through a hellish fire swamp. Things have settled down now. As of the writing of this book, Pam is fifty-seven, at the finale of perimenopause, with some minor symptoms. Julie is a sixty-one-year-old, full-fledged member of the menopausal club. The last couple of years were intensely stressful for her and activated a few of her symptoms again. Most midlife women have a ton on their beautiful shoulders (work, kids, aging parents, shifting relationships, and more) along with a body that is going through hormonal chaos. At times, we didn't think we would make it to the other side. Our wish for you is that you can have peace in your body, that you can choose a healthcare routine that supports you and brings balance to your hormones, and that you can shine with more confidence, embracing your wisdom and ageless beauty.

So What Is Happening With Your Hormones?

Refresher: Perimenopause can begin fifteen years before the onset of menopause, with predictably declining levels of progesterone followed by wildly fluctuating levels of estrogen and ending with a significant drop in estrogen. Perimenopause and the early years of menopause are a crucial time for focusing on our long-term health, even if we are symptom-free. These years seem to be an inflection point, and even small health problems should be considered and managed. Your body is going through major changes. To have a gentler menopausal experience, as well as to prevent future health issues that could be more serious, make self-care a priority.

Don't Ignore Your Symptoms

Even as the information out there is getting clearer and more of us are sharing our wisdom, experiences, and solutions, it is still the *dark ages* of menopause. We have been doing some serious digging regarding hormone balance for the past fifteen years so that we can support our clients, friends, and ourselves. We have our hearts and minds focused on menopause, and thankfully, new insights and beneficial data are arriving daily. But this can also make it difficult to discern what is true and what the best answers are for us to create a more positive midlife journey. Educating yourself will help you to be prepared and will help you advocate for your needs during perimenopause and menopause.

FEMALE HORMONAL DECLINE GRAPH[39]

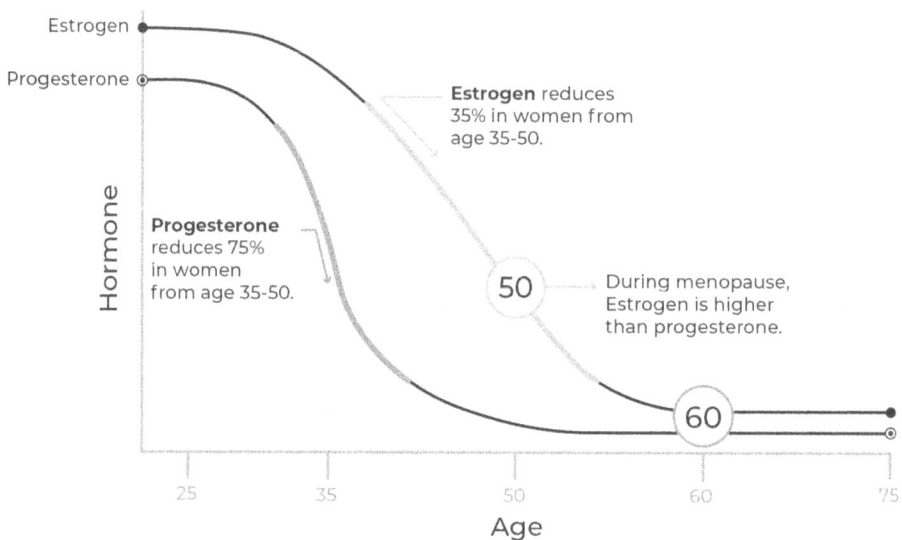

While the above graph is an oversimplified example of the hormonal decline during perimenopause, the amazing Dr. Sharon Malone, gynecologist and author of *Grown Woman Talk* has a deeper explanation of what is happening during this time. She says, "There is not a straight line in the decline of your hormones during perimenopause. Unlike men, whose testosterone levels decline with age in a gentler fashion, our hormone levels fluctuate wildly during this period. Your estrogen levels can be too high one day, only to plummet the next. Your brain and body are in a constant state of recalibration in response to these hormonal shifts."[40]

Let's start with some basics about female hormones. Hormones are messengers that manage different functions in our body and communicate with our muscles, and skeletal tissues and organs such as our skin, brain and endocrine glands. They have a huge impact on our moods and behavior as well as a host of physiological functions. Any imbalance or decrease in the appropriate level of hormones in our bodies can affect our physical, emotional, and mental health. Hormones are necessary for the health of our bodies! The primary sex steroid hormones for women are estrogen, progesterone, testosterone and DHEA.

Estrogen

If you feel like you are losing some of your mojo, estrogen is the primary hormone that helps us feel confident and sensual! Remember how you felt when you were sixteen and some hot human walked by? And all those young girls screaming and fainting during Beatles concerts? That is some hyped-up estrogen. We also refer to estrogen as the "tend and befriend" hormone. If you have seen the movie *Barbie*, Barbieland was all about women tending and befriending. Estrogen is one of the factors that supports us in creating deep and long-lasting friendship bonds.

There are several types of estrogen. Estradiol has over 300 roles in the body and supports female organs, including the uterus, vagina, breasts, and bladder, as well as the health of our bones, brain, and cardiovascular system.[41] There are estrogen receptors in every organ in the body. We may have relatively optimal levels during early perimenopause. As perimenopause moves along, our levels decrease, and symptoms such as hot flashes, night sweats, brain fog, vaginal dryness, joint pain, heart palpitations, and more may begin to appear and increase.

In her book, *The New Menopause*, Dr. Mary Claire Haver explains why estrogen is so important for women's health. "Estrogen isn't just a pretty hormone that's key to reproductive capabilities; it's responsible for so much more. There are estrogen receptors throughout almost every organ system in your body, and as your levels drop, these cells begin to lose their ability to assist in maintaining your health in other areas, including your heart, cognitive function, bone integrity, and blood sugar balance."[42]

Fun fact: Midlife men have more estrogen in their bodies than menopausal women! Something to think about.[43]

Progesterone

Progesterone is produced in the ovaries and adrenals, and its main functions are to support the menstrual cycle and pregnancy. It is the calming hormone that helps us stay cool and collected. It helps mitigate night sweats, promotes deep sleep, and is a natural antidepressant. As perimenopause begins, progesterone will decline faster than estrogen. This imbalance can contribute to the symptoms of irritability, anxiety, and yes, *rage*—as if we don't have enough reasons to be angry.

Symptoms of **declining progesterone** can also include:

- Worsening PMS
- Unexplained weight gain
- Disrupted and/or poor sleep
- Sore or swollen breasts
- Bloating in the belly and/or ankles
- Unusually heavy or painful periods
- Miscarriage in the first trimester
- And again, recurring headaches

Progesterone is also needed to balance the effects of estrogen. So when progesterone is out of balance, you may experience estrogen dominance, which is essentially *too much* estrogen relative to progesterone.

Symptoms of **estrogen dominance**:

- Low sex drive
- Weight gain (again!)
- Irregular periods
- Bloating
- Hot flashes
- Insomnia
- Brain fog
- Gallbladder problems
- Anxiety or depression

- Fibrocystic lumps in the breasts
- Mood swings
- Increased breast size

Testosterone

Testosterone is mainly produced in the ovaries and supports libido big time, as well as strong bones and muscle tone. Testosterone has been genderized as a male hormone, but the truth is it's an androgen that every vertebrate animal produces. In fact, when we share that women have more testosterone in their bodies than estrogen, most women are shocked. But, yes, it's true! In women, testosterone is converted into estradiol, which is one of the most potent types of estrogen. Unfortunately, not many doctors are educated about how important testosterone is in the female body.

When testosterone levels fall, we may experience loss of interest in sex, weight gain (particularly belly fat), lack of drive, muscle atrophy, and decreased cognitive functioning—yup, that's brain fog. Prescribing testosterone therapy for women remains controversial. Some women enjoy additional testosterone when using hormone therapy, and other women may start manifesting the symptoms of excess testosterone, like thinning hair, an increase in facial hair, and possibly aggressive behavior. As no two women are alike, it is very important to individualize the approach to hormone restoration.

Symptoms of **low testosterone** may also include:

- Low libido
- Difficulty reaching orgasm
- Unexplained or severe fatigue
- Severe brain fog; feeling like the brain doesn't work
- Loss of muscle mass/decreased response to exercise

- Fat around the waist and hips
- Increased feelings of sadness

2002 Women's Health Initiative Study

Let's address the controversial 2002 study that, for the past twenty years, has caused confusion within the medical community and created a shroud over hormone therapy (HT) for women. Interestingly, by the '70s, HT was the standard treatment for the ailments of menopause. According to the National Institutes of Health, back in 1975, synthetic estrogen was the fifth most prescribed drug in the United States. Even into the '80s and '90s, it was fairly common for women of menopausal age to be prescribed HT.[44] Around 2003, Julie remembers meeting a very lively, much older woman who shared with her that she had been on HT for years and didn't give a damn about the recent studies. She had been on HT for a couple of decades, felt great, and planned to do so until she died.

"HRT is not perfect, but it has suffered from a bad reputation." In 2002, the Women's Health Initiative (WHI) study made news when it suggested that "HRT might increase the risk of breast cancer and doctors began shying away from prescribing it. Unfortunately, the study had design flaws that led to incorrect conclusions about HRT, and those misperceptions were amplified and widely reported by the media, leading to widespread misinformation."[45]

The WHI studied the protective effects of estrogen on heart disease to see if it could demonstrate that fewer women would die of heart disease if they were using estrogen. The women in the study were started on synthetic estrogen. Their average age was sixty-three, having gone through menopause around ten to fifteen years earlier. Many of the women in the study were not only well beyond menopause, but many were also obese, and over half of them were former or current smokers—both of which are significant cancer risks. The women were being prescribed Premarin (derived from pregnant mare urine) or Prempro (a combination of Premarin and a synthetic progestin). Not exactly bio-identical! The study was halted after a minimal increased risk of breast cancer, heart disease, blood clots, and stroke were found.[46]

The medical community became terrified to offer estrogen as a solution to their patients, even though they had known for years that it was the best treatment for mood changes, poor sleep, and hot flashes. In the United States, prescriptions dropped by 70% and by 66% in the United Kingdom.[47][48]

One of the principal investigators of the WHI study, Professor Emeritus of Family Medicine and Public Health at the University of California, Robert D. Langer, MD, MPH, is quoted as saying, "I believe that women who have gone through menopause since the WHI report have been harmed, and in many cases left to suffer in poor health because of the unwarranted degree of fear stoked by the WHI. Not all women have indications for HRT, but for those who do and who initiate *within* ten years of menopause, benefits are both short-term (relieving hot flashes and painful intercourse) and long-term (bone health, coronary heart disease risk reduction). It's time to get past the misinformation and hysteria generated by the irregular circumstances of the WHI report and stop denying potential benefits to women who have indications and may be helped."[49]

Dr. Kelly Casperson, a brilliant and humorous urologist and sex educator, and the author of *You Are Not Broken,* says, "It's taken twenty years for this conversation to get back to the facts: hormones are life-improving and very safe for many women. Estrogen (especially when given in young menopause) protects against heart disease, anxiety and depression, breast cancer, colon cancer, cognitive problems, insulin resistance, and osteoporosis. Several studies have shown hormone replacement increases longevity." She also shares that without hormones, vulvovaginal atrophy occurs in fifty to 80% of menopausal women.[50]

For over fifteen years, we have done our research on the 2002 Women's Health Initiative study. We have read about the inaccuracies of the study, listened to lectures at health care conferences on the benefits of HT, and spoken with many, many MDs and asked them their thoughts. Interestingly, a study of female OB/GYNs in midlife revealed that the majority of those surveyed used HT themselves even though they were not recommending it to their patients![51]

In February 2023, twenty years after the WHI study, Susan Dominus wrote an outstanding article in *The New York Times Magazine* that went viral.[52] It was about the risks and the benefits of HT, reviewing the 2002 study, "Women Have Been Misled About Menopause." It is worth quoting some powerful responses from her readers:

One said, "This article touches on the grief I still feel after leaving a job that I loved at 53 . . . I asked for a sabbatical and was turned down . . . It didn't occur to me to ask for medical leave. This article gives me hope for women. Bringing light to the shame, the darkness, and the cultural misogyny around menopause is a good thing. At one point, I said to my husband: 'No wonder they called us witches. Anyone who survives this has to be magical.'"

Another said, "I worked through two pregnancies, pumped breast milk for years in a bathroom stall, and juggled child care schedules. Pregnancy and small children couldn't defeat me. Menopause did. I would sit in meetings stressed out that I was going to leave a puddle of blood in the meeting room chair. I couldn't sleep. I bled for months. I'm on hormone therapy now, but I'm stressed out about retirement because of the terrible damage I did to my career and salary when I quit my job at the height of my earning power."

And another: "I'm taking this article to my next OBGYN appointment. The doctors at my women's center (even the young female doctors) act like I'm ridiculous to ask about HRT. Thanks for this article. The medical community treats menopausal women like they're invisible."

In 2014, The American College of Obstetrics and Gynecology (ACOG) made its position on hormone therapy clear. "Systemic estrogen therapy (with or without progestin) has been shown to be the best treatment for hot flashes and night sweats. Both systemic and local estrogen therapy relieve vaginal dryness. Systemic estrogen protects against the bone loss that occurs early in menopause. This can help prevent osteoporosis."[53]

While discussing the WHI study and HT for menopausal women,

Peter Attia, MD, held nothing back when he said, "Hands down the biggest screw-up in the medical field in the last 25 years."[54]

Considering Hormone Therapy

What was formerly referred to as hormone replacement therapy (HRT) is now known as hormone therapy (HT) or menopause hormone therapy (MHT). Hormone *replacement* therapy implies that hormones need to be replaced due to a medical problem and that menopause is a disease. Menopause is biologically normal—even though it may not feel that way!

Outstanding OB/GYN Suzanne Gilberg, author of *Menopause Bootcamp*, recently shared in *Glamour* magazine, " . . . I oppose the pathologizing of perimenopause and menopause. The menopausal transition is clinically defined as a physiological change, not a disease requiring diagnosis. This distinction is important because all women deserve management, education, and support from their health care providers, regardless of what testing results indicate.

"It's time to talk to your doctor if you experience any disruption in your life. Don't feel like you need to grin and bear it or suffer in silence—that is an outdated narrative that keeps women's needs in the shadows. Instead, I want women to embrace the menopause transition as an opportunity to live out loud with life, joy, and support."[55] Love it!

If you decide to choose HT, the first ten years of menopause are the most critical. However, your practitioner may recommend you begin during perimenopause to alleviate your symptoms. Since each one of us is bio-individual, you are entitled to a treatment plan that addresses your unique concerns and desires for your lifestyle. HT is not a one-size-fits-all treatment, and tweaking your treatment is often necessary. HT is available in patches, pills, creams, gels, lozenges, implants, and suppositories. You can choose either FDA-approved synthetic hormones, bioidentical hormones, or compounded bioidentical hormones. In the United Kingdom, bioidentical hormones are referred to as "body identical." Bioidentical and body identical hormones are man-made hormones derived from plants that are chemically identical to those the human body produces. Most of the physicians we have spoken with agree that estrogen HT should *not* be taken orally, even though oral formulations are still available. However, we do have friends who have used oral progesterone very successfully. Again, your care should be customized with your trusted providers.

Hormone Therapy does a lot more than just relieve hot flashes and night sweats. It can relieve anxiety, depression, brain fog, vaginal dryness, low libido, and sleep issues as well as offer the long-term, beneficial effects of lowering the risk of certain cancers, osteoporosis, heart disease, and dementia.

Many studies indicate that estrogen preserves cognitive function and may delay or prevent the onset of Alzheimer's disease. The decline in estrogen during menopause directly correlates with the onset of osteoporosis. Women lose around 10% of their bone mass in the first five years after menopause.[56] Research has shown that estradiol (the most common form of estrogen used for HT) is the key hormonal regulator of bone metabolism in women and men. Estradiol concentrations can correlate with and predict the risk of fractures. Post-menopausal women using estradiol have a greater muscle-building response with exercise. Estradiol contributes to an increase of collagen and elastin content in the tendons and ligaments, improving strength.[57][58] Post-menopause, cardiovascular disease increases significantly. Lab studies have shown that estradiol has significant cardiovascular protective effects.[59]

Most women don't learn about perimenopause and menopause until they're already experiencing symptoms—symptoms that can become unbearable before hormone therapy (HT) is even considered. Yet we aspire to live purposeful, passionate lives beyond menopause, and the choices we make during this transition can shape our health and well-being for decades to come. That's why it's so important to be proactive—and we're here to support you in making these years your best yet.

Let us be super clear here: We are pro-woman and pro-you, whether or not your experience of caring for yourself during menopause includes HT. We are offering this information regarding HT so that you can be better informed about the choices you make to support yourself during the menopausal transition.

We have friends and clients who have chosen, for a variety of reasons, not to use HT. Some have family histories of cancer or have personally had female cancers, such as breast, ovarian, and uterine cancer. In an article from the Cleveland Clinic regarding estrogen-dependent cancers, "Experts know that *several* different factors play a role in turning healthy cells cancerous. When these factors are present, estrogen can act as a spark."[60]

We also have family, friends, and clients who have chosen not to use HT because they feel pretty great and are relatively symptom-free. But they do attend to their health, have healthy lifestyles, use supplements, have regular checkups and blood tests, and have done their research. HT is not appropriate for all women, and you must review the risks and benefits with a trustworthy, experienced menopause practitioner and do your research to determine what is the best treatment for *your* menopausal journey.

We have also been very fortunate to be friends with many female health care practitioners and physicians who have a deep concern for the health and well-being of their patients, and they continue to dive deeply into the latest research so that they can offer the highest level of care and service. HT has been a powerful journey of discovery for both of us, providing a clear path to wellness.

JULIE

Around 2005, when I was in my early forties and struggling to heal my autoimmune issue, I did a lot of reading and research on using hormone therapy to address health challenges. I then consulted with a highly recommended physician who reviewed my bloodwork and prescribed bioidentical oral estrogen capsules and progesterone lozenges.

It was the beginning of a wild ride. While taking the hormones, I experienced a lot of anger. We went on a beautiful family vacation in Turks and Caicos, and I thought, "If I can't feel happy here in this incredible place, when will I ever be able to feel happiness?" I felt bloated, plus I had intense reactions to many foods and constant digestive upset. I couldn't think clearly, and then the physician prescribed Lexapro for me in addition to the HT I was already taking. He told me it would help further with my estrogen deficiency. I wondered, "How does that work? An antidepressant to address estrogen deficiency?" Taking the medication like a "good" patient made my symptoms even worse. He also suggested a whole slew of supplements (twenty-six to be exact), none of which were cracking the code.

Looking back, it's shocking that I agreed to this course of treatment. I just didn't know what I didn't know, and I was desperate. It is even more shocking that this was an acceptable protocol being prescribed by a supposedly excellent health care provider!

After around six months of using HT, I started having horrible pain on my right side. I thought maybe it was my liver, and I ended up on the bathroom floor in excruciating pain, unable to breathe. The pain passed, and then I started to turn yellow. Eyes yellow. Skin yellow. Jaundice. I ended up having two emergency surgeries, one to remove gallstones that had lodged in my bile duct and the other to remove my gallbladder, because I had developed a five-centimeter gallstone. And guess what? Estrogen taken orally can contribute to the formation of gallstones! Thankfully, oral estrogen is rarely prescribed anymore due to advances in patches, creams, and suppositories. I stopped using the HT immediately and classified it in the "never again" category.

Then ten years passed, and well, "never say never." I cleaned up my health even further, healed my autoimmune disease, and did the work to address some of the root causes that were taking my body offline. I was now using only a few cutting-edge supplements that provided cellular detoxification for toxins (environmental, heavy metals, etc.) and hormone balancing, recommended by an excellent MD, PhD, and happily sleeping like a baby. The depression had lifted, and even my fibrocystic breast disease was resolved. Around fifty-one, I began talking to more doctors, reading more, and realizing that maybe, just *maybe*, I should reconsider HT.

I also had a few wake-up calls: three minor car accidents. No one was hurt, and there was very little damage. In the third accident, I'd been looking out my car window while driving, checking out a fabulous skirt in a store window, and rear-ended the car in front of me. After that, I realized my brain just felt funky, seemed to skip a beat, and I would space out. My insurance agent said she noticed she gets a lot of claims from menopausal women who are in car accidents. No comment!

I realized I was doing everything I could to address my menopausal issues, and it wasn't doing the trick. With the support of an outstanding female physician who is an expert in bioidentical hormone replacement, I began using topical hormone creams daily. I have been using them for over ten years and am in excellent health. Sure, I wish I had the sharp brain function and stamina of my twenty-five-year-old self, but hey, I am happy to be alive, strong, and symptom-free. Regarding sharp brain function, I believe that my intuition, elder wisdom, and life experiences have begun to take up more space in my brain!

US

As women, many of us are very familiar with the runaround, lack of compassionate care, and generally ineffective, or worse—dangerous—guidance that we experience with our health issues. Both of us have stories from clients that are heartbreaking. This can be even more challenging during perimenopause and menopause, as fewer than one in five OB/GYN medical students receive training in menopausal medicine.[61] Unfortunately, most visits with our physicians don't allow sufficient time to discuss the challenges we may be having, with some appointments only lasting ten minutes maximum. Typically, this is due to insurance constraints. Additionally, according to a Harris Poll, one in three women aged forty-five to fifty-four are given an incorrect diagnosis when experiencing the challenges of menopause.[62] We hold the hope that menopause will eventually become a medical specialty. Women deserve *so* much better!

PAM

I'm huge on doing everything as naturally as possible, and thought I would cruise through menopause "naturally." However, when I was in my mid-forties and started experiencing insomnia, night sweats, brain fog, rage (yes, real rage), and crazy weight gain, I was willing to take anything that would make me feel better—or at least like my normal self. Oh, and by the way, I was still having regular periods, every twenty-eight days to the day. So, clearly, I must have been in perimenopause but didn't know it.

I initially talked to my OB/GYN back in 2018 at my annual appointment and shared the symptoms I was having. While she lent me a sympathetic ear, she dismissed the idea that I was anywhere near menopause because I was still having regular periods. She told me I was most likely suffering from depression, gave me a prescription for Wellbutrin (an antidepressant), and told me to talk to a therapist. I didn't take the antidepressants because I didn't feel depressed, and intuitively, I felt like my symptoms were hormonal. So I continued to tough it out for a couple of years, thinking I would eventually feel better.

In early 2020, I felt like my brain went completely offline. Intuitively, I thought it had something to do with hormones, so I found a doctor who was familiar with bioidentical hormones. I did a complete hormone panel, which confirmed my suspicions that I had a hormone issue. I had extremely low testosterone, almost non-existent. I knew enough to know low testosterone was most likely contributing to my brain fog and weight gain, plus a lack of muscle tone despite regular weight training. This doctor prescribed bioidentical testosterone for me, which I used diligently as directed for around six months. At first, I had energy and felt great. Until I didn't. Night sweats came back in full force, and I still wasn't losing any weight. I was also super crabby. And rageful. And still having regular periods.

In late 2020, I started having what I thought were chest pains. My heart felt like it was beating out of my chest, and I couldn't catch my breath. Heart problems run in my family, so my husband immediately whisked me off to the ER. They took me very seriously and admitted me. After four days of blood work, stress tests, an angiogram and multiple ECGs that showed I had the heart of an athlete (!), a female cardiologist suggested what I was feeling might be heart palpitations, a symptom of perimenopause. I had no idea!

Frantically searching for answers, I then found another doctor who told me to stop the testosterone and put me on a static dose of bioidentical estradiol and progesterone. Well, I still felt like complete garbage. Plus, I wasn't sleeping, my brain was completely offline, I had horrible gut issues and crazy heart palpitations, and I found myself raging (again) in Whole Foods because there were no ripe avocados. I was at my wit's end!

Desperate to crack the hormone code, I finally found a doctor who put me on physiologic hormone restoration, a bioidentical plant-based estradiol and progesterone with non-static dosages that follow the lunar cycle. Within a couple of months, I started to sleep, had fewer mood swings, no rage, and more energy.

However, around six months in, I started losing my energy and brain again. What the hell?! I had more lab work done, and it showed, once again, that I had extremely low testosterone. Now I have added a low dose of testosterone to my hormone therapy, and not only is my brain back online, but my energy is back, my heart palpitations are gone, and I can see some muscle tone from all the exercise I do. (P.S. My husband is elated my libido is back—and so am I!) Hormone therapy has completely changed my quality of life.

Us

In *You Are Not Broken*, Dr. Kelly Casperson says, "What about the thought that 'menopause is natural' and you shouldn't take anything for it? My response is, if you want to be all-natural, don't have air conditioning. Don't wear shoes. Get rid of your car. You can't have modern conveniences and then tell people you shouldn't have vaginal estrogen. What I want is for you to know that you've been sold a pack of lies about hormones that are just as big as the ones society taught you about sex."[63]

We are very aware that some of the information we have shared regarding HT remains controversial and is constantly being revised and updated. But when women share about their menopausal journey, shattering taboos, we all rise. We need a universal standard of care, more research, far more and improved education for health care providers, and many more women's voices supporting one another. Let's all help each other crack the code on menopause. We have to end this suffering!

"It's amazing how many opinions are out there about what women should and shouldn't do with our bodies, and how much pain we ought to endure ... that don't come from women themselves. As delivery vessels for the species, we've been considered common property since time began. Decisions about what is and isn't best for us have, for thousands of years, been made by people with an entirely different perspective, plus a penis."[64]

To receive the best care possible, we recommend you begin tracking your symptoms. It's very important to be prepared for your appointment with a practitioner with menopause experience. Consider making a separate appointment so that you have time just to discuss your symptoms. Bring a list of your health issues and questions, and if your practitioner says anything dismissive or behaves as if they know your body better than you do, consider finding someone who will support you! Again, through most labs now, you can also order your blood work, and we have many clients and friends who choose to do that. (It's also a way to get around any insurance issues that your provider may have regarding ordering certain blood panels that might not be covered.)

It is very disturbing to us, and to many of our clients, that insurance companies don't often cover appointments with many practitioners who are qualified in menopausal care and that essential, comprehensive blood tests and other diagnostic tests are often an additional charge. Unfortunately, bioidentical hormone therapy is not usually covered either. We partner with practitioners who are very understanding of these issues and choose to keep their pricing reasonable.

Questions To Ask Your Health Care Practitioners

Here are some questions we have asked of our health care providers and physicians. We encourage our clients to ask the questions that apply to them:

- What are your thoughts about HT? What is your experience of using HT with your patients? What would you do for *your* health?
- Is HT the right next step for me? And what is the diagnostic process for that? (Labs, tests?)

- With a family history of breast cancer, what do you suggest I do to manage my menopausal symptoms?

- What supplements are you using to support your patients' hormonal balance and long-term wellness?

- I've read that environmental toxins can disrupt endocrine function, causing hormonal imbalance and perhaps contributing to disease. Do you have recommendations on how I can address this?

- I have been gaining weight, and my eating habits and exercise routine haven't changed. Why is this happening, and what lifestyle choices would you recommend?

- I am crying a lot, getting angered by the smallest things, and feeling more vulnerable to stress. What might be causing this, and what are some solutions?

- I am not sleeping well, and I wake up often in the middle of the night with anxiety. Other than medication, what steps can I take to improve my sleep and get deep rest?

- I have hot flashes and night sweats. Is there something I can do or take to mitigate them?

- My libido is vanishing, and sex is painful. I've heard about testosterone, vaginal estrogen, Addyi, lube, and lasers. What steps can I take to restore my sex drive and enjoy sex again?

- When I sneeze or exercise, I lose urine. Do you know of pelvic-floor exercises or other therapies that would be helpful? What's the latest research on lasers to help with incontinence? Does HT help with this?

- I would like to measure my bone density. At what age should I get a DEXA scan?

Blood Tests

The following are essential blood tests to have a comprehensive assessment of your health. These are very important whether you are thinking about choosing HT or not. You can request these from your physician. If you have excellent insurance, all of these may be covered. Please check in with your doctor first. Additionally, there are now labs where you can order the blood work for yourself online and have a phlebotomist come to your home. You will have to pay directly—no insurance—but often, they can be much less expensive than co-pays or out-of-network costs.

- All hormone levels (If you are menstruating, day 12 or day 21)
- Hormone panel: estradiol, estrone, progesterone, DHEA-S, SHBG, cortisol, total testosterone, free testosterone, luteinizing hormone (LH), follicle-stimulating hormone (FSH), IGF-1
- CBC with differential
- Comprehensive metabolic panel
- Thyroid panel: TSH, Free T3, Free T4, Reverse T3
- Lipid panel: HDL, LDL, triglycerides (TRG), total cholesterol
- Iron panel
- Autoimmune markers
- Inflammatory / Cardiac risk factors: hs-CRP, ApoB, lipoprotein (a)
- ALT and AST
- Homocysteine
- Blood Glucose Levels

- Hemoglobin A1C
- Magnesium
- Vitamin D
- Vitamin B12
- Uric acid

Gentle Recommendations for Balancing Your Hormones (Whether You Choose to Use HT or Not):

- Eat nutrient-dense, low-sugar, whole foods. Research shows that an anti-inflammatory, plant-based food plan is very healing and promotes longevity. It's been our experience that we feel happier and have more mental clarity and energy when we eat this way most of the time!

- Reduce the toxic load in your life. Drink filtered water, and, if you can, shower with filtered water. Our skin is our largest eliminative organ—so it's great if you can use a shower filter. Have a high-quality air purifier in your living and sleeping spaces. Avoid plastics, including water bottles. This is beneficial for our environment, too.

- Ideally, get eight or more hours of sleep per night. Take a high-quality magnesium glycinate supplement before bedtime. Have a sleep routine. Visit the QR code to view our sleep routine document.

- Move your body every day. Enjoy walking, yoga, swimming, and strength training. Many apps offer great exercise programs.

- Drink half your body weight (in pounds) in ounces of water daily. Add lemon, limes, or oranges—and we often add an electrolyte powder to our water, especially on days we exercise. It helps with dehydration big time, and we seem to need more hydration with menopause.

- Treat yourself to Epsom salt baths before bed. Make this special. Add wonderfully smelling essential oils. This will help to gently detoxify your body and encourage relaxation.

- Getting morning sunshine will support your circadian rhythm and will help with happiness and sleep, too! Consider investing in a light lamp for the dark winter months.

- Stress is a killer, and it's challenging to balance your hormones if your body is in fight-or-flight with your nervous system jacked up. Start your morning with gratitude, put on a happy song and dance, meditate, write in a journal, or pray. Then take time during the day to love yourself.

- Take a multivitamin for women in midlife. Some include fantastic herbs that support symptoms. And make sure you are getting enough of vitamins D3, K, B's, and C, omega-3, and zinc. Blood testing panels will reveal any deficiencies. (See the resources for our recommendations for supplements and testing options by visiting the QR code at the beginning or end of the book.)

- Spend time with women friends who love and support you! If you are shifting away from friends who aren't moving in your direction, be gentle with yourself and take the time to invite new friends into your life who enjoy being with you in this next phase of life. True support from like-minded friends is priceless.

- Reconnect with your cultural and personal identity as well. Go deep. Feel who you truly are beyond your body and its evolving needs.

Busting Menopausal Myths

- **It's the same for everyone:** Not by a long shot. In speaking with women, we have heard varying symptoms—to none at all. Menopause is not a one-size-fits-all, and every woman's experience is unique.

1. **Menopause means weight gain:** Not necessarily. Sex hormones, cortisol, and lifestyle choices all play a role here, and as we age, controlling weight can be more challenging. It is essential to exercise regularly, eat healthy foods, and practice self-care.

2. **I don't have perimenopause symptoms, so my menopause will be a breeze:** Sorry ladies, just because you lucked out during perimenopause doesn't mean you get off easy. Some women only have symptoms during menopause. But if you are mindful of your health and wellness, you will likely have a gentler menopause.

3. **Menopause starts at age fifty:** Fifty-one is the average age, and women can go into menopause as early as their thirties and as late as their mid to late fifties. As a result of chemotherapy or surgery, the ovaries may stop functioning (medical menopause), and these women may experience the same symptoms as women in natural menopause, or they might be more severe due to the abrupt onset of menopause.

4. **I just have a few symptoms, so I'm probably okay:** It's important to discuss all of your symptoms with a healthcare practitioner. Perimenopause and menopause symptoms can mask other serious health issues.

5. **Now that I'm in menopause, I feel like I'm over the hill:** Hey, let's consider ourselves to be better than ever. You are a goddess. Claim your wisdom and all of your life experience.

The young ones may have glowier skin, but believe it: You are entering your golden years. This is a time of life to celebrate.

6. **My sex drive will disappear:** Perhaps not! Some women report a strong libido after menopause due to being empty nesters and no longer worrying about pregnancy. And we have an entire chapter dedicated to reclaiming your sexuality in midlife!

7. **I'm all alone:** No, you're not. That's why we wrote this book and created our coaching program. We wanted to be a source of support and education for women.

Our message to you, dear reader—don't give up! Both of us had to search to find the right team to help us navigate this journey, and we can assure you that there are plenty of caring, knowledgeable, and compassionate healthcare providers who will listen and do their best to support you, too. Whether you choose to use HT or not, you have the right to choose. And be open to new information—as more women are getting involved in the conversation, more information is coming to light, and many communities are popping up, like ours. Let's change the conversation for midlife women together!

CHAPTER 4

TURN YOURSELF ON

Reviewed by Vesna Skul, MD, FACP

"You are like menopause in a snowsuit. Hotter than hell!"
—Naughty Betty

*"I'm going through perimenopause at the moment.
It is really bizarre, but it is the most glorious invitation into
a new season and chapter in my life . . . I'm the sexiest I've ever been.
And when I say that, I mean I feel the most myself . . .
I'm going to be sexy all over the place. Living my life with my juice."*
—Tracee Ellis Ross

"Every desire of your body is holy."
—Rumi

For centuries, men have been the ones telling the story of female sexuality. Penis envy—need we say more? Only very recently, studies conducted by leading female scientists in the fields of human sexuality and women's reproductive health have discovered that women's desire is often measured incorrectly.[65] It is now understood that arousal for women likely depends on their erotic relationships with themselves. Dr. Meredith

Chivers, founder and director of Queen's University Sexuality and Gender Laboratory, has shared, "It's frustrating to hear it repeated over and over again that men have stronger (libidos) than women do as if it's a simple fact."[66] Our sexual desire starts with ourselves, our relationship to our bodies, and our experience of our pleasure. Indeed, midlife can be the time to fall in love with ourselves.

Julie

During the final years of my marriage, while I was in menopause, my sexuality had completely fallen apart. I felt like I was withering away. I saw my future if this continued, and it did not look good. While discussing this with my best friend from college, she remarked that I was the most sexual person she knew. While I accepted it as a beautiful affirmation and certainly knew myself to be *sensual* internally, I wondered, "Really? What does *that* even mean?"

I had always been a serial monogamist who loved very deeply and invested fully in my relationships, but over the years, I had come to believe that I was "too much"—and not just in the bedroom. I absorbed myself in other interests, thinking that maybe if I changed in some way, tried harder, or improved any number of things, my partner might become more interested in me sexually. I had a lot of shame around my longing for more intimacy. I had a lot of shame around my longing for more passion. I had a lot of shame about my sexuality. I didn't even know how much shame there was . . . or what I was truly longing for in a love relationship.

Things began to unravel in my consciousness. To reconnect with my body and reclaim myself and my sexuality, I embarked on a midlife journey of rediscovering myself as a woman. I began reading books, doing research, and attending seminars, classes, and retreats about women's power, trauma, sexuality, the female brain, patriarchy, and cliteracy—oh yes, *clitoral literacy*—and I even took a class called "Vaginal Kung Fu." Certainly, some of it was way out there. But what I longed for was calling to me: I desired more.

In Regena Thomashauer's book *Pussy: A Reclamation*, she writes, "We don't realize that it's our enjoyment of ourselves and our bodies that creates, and re-creates, radiance inside of us. The last place we are taught to look for our turn-on is our own bodies. Yet a woman who is turned on to herself and her life is a woman in her highest power. Being turned on is a spiritual state. It is the golden thread that connects a woman to the meaning of her life and to her desire."[67] I began to do the transformational work of reclaiming myself.

Let's face it—as women, many of us have been socialized to hide our pain and keep our "dark and dirty" stuff to ourselves. Don't be too sexual, but don't be too modest either. Express big emotions, and we're called *hysterical*. (We despise that word. It originates from the Greek *hystera*, implying that due to our anatomy, women are inherently irrational and overly emotional. And an unbelievable fact: The term "female hysteria" was not removed from the DSM, the Diagnostic and Statistical Manual of Mental Disorders, until 1980.)[68] And it's often uncommon for women to feel safe speaking openly about sexual dissatisfaction. If we do, the response may be minimizing: "What's the big deal?" or "Is it really that important?"

Dr. Kelly Casperson nails it. "We care about men's pleasure and not women's pleasure. We call women who enjoy sex dirty words. The woman is always the problem when it comes to a desire mismatch: If her desire is too high, that's her problem. If her desire is too low, that's her problem. The system is broken, yet most of us are left feeling like *we* are broken."[69]

Then when we enter perimenopause, that's often when the shit hits the fan. Something's got to give. And since more women are waking up in their forties, fifties, and sixties, we are beginning to see that something different, something more enlivening, might be possible for us. Friends are leaving unhappy partnerships and marriages, they are no longer willing to tolerate abusive co-workers and toxic work cultures, or they just want a deeper level of fulfillment.

Desires, including sexual desires, that we may have dreamed of in our twenties resurface. We may have a longing for a bigger love story, to be treated with dignity and respect, to have honest and authentic friendships, and to feel the call to be truly alive. As we know, many of us, in order to survive, may have suppressed our trauma and our losses and lived with self-blame and self-hate. We may feel unable to even imagine living full, creative lives defined by love and deep sexual satisfaction.

Every woman that we have ever spoken with has experienced gender-based difficulties or abuse, and as we all know, women around the world have experienced unbelievable horror. So very many of us, and generations before us, have experienced the rupture of sexual assault, profound loss, and the death of dreams and desires—all included in what Regena Thomashauer refers to as the 4 Ds: devastation, despair, disenfranchisement, and depression. We can remain there, in some version of the 4 Ds, for all of our lives. It can manifest as severe mental or physical illness, toxic work environments, unhappy and unhealthy relationships, and more.

Ignoring our sexuality can be like amputating a part of ourselves—even if we may have been ignoring it for most of our lives. We have been conditioned by a patriarchal world culture, after all. And it starts early; only half of all Americans receive sex education before they are eighteen years old.[70] We don't even realize what we're missing. Our brief sex ed in school was all about pregnancy prevention—not about our pleasure preservation! And we are certain that there was no mention of the clitoris.

Pam

I have faced numerous assaults, more than I can count. Sadly, it's my experience that most of the women I know have also been assaulted in some way, shape, or form. I vividly recall an encounter at twenty-one as a college student at a bar with friends. A guy came up to me, callously grabbed both of my breasts, and said, "Tuning in to Radio Europe." I was completely shocked, and my knee-jerk reaction was to give him a swift kick in the balls. He then called me a bitch (the nerve!). Seriously, I could not believe someone would do something like that to me.

A few years later, I was twenty-four, out of college, and working in downtown Chicago. I ventured out for lunch and still remember clearly what I was wearing—a shortish (but not mini) black flippy skirt and chunky black sandals. Out of nowhere, a man approached me from behind, lifted my skirt, and grabbed my butt. I screamed in complete shock and ran after him (as did several people who had seen what happened), but he ran down some stairs and got away.

At twenty-five, I was living in an apartment in what I thought was a safe neighborhood. A key was needed to open the front door, and visitors had to be buzzed in. I had come home rather early from a birthday party, between 8:30 and 9:00 p.m. Unbeknownst to me, a man pushed his way in behind me in an attempt to rape me in the entryway. I had to pee so badly, and I pleaded with him to just let me pee. Finally, I threatened to pee on him, and he let me go. Fortunately, that man ended up being caught for assaulting multiple women. I was able to ID him in a lineup, and he ended up serving time in prison. Another year, another assault.

These experiences, among others, have marked me profoundly, revealing a distressing pattern far too many women share. I am aware my own stories are just one thread among the countless others who have suffered similar indignities. It's time for change, a collective awakening that refuses to have these stories remain silent. By sharing our stories, our truths, we have the power to show the reality that assaults, physical *and* verbal, aren't just isolated incidents but part of the gendered violence that has been ignored for too long.

As I got older, I recognized trust, vulnerability, and intimacy were areas where I struggled in past relationships, and it became clear these were issues I needed to address. Cognitive behavior therapy was instrumental for me in overcoming the impact of assault trauma. With therapy, I was able to heal my trauma, reclaim my sexual health, and take back my power. I am now in a loving, happy, and healthy marriage with a man who not only values me but is supportive of my healing and growth. And, in my fifties, I am enjoying the best sex of my life!

Julie

While reading *Pussy*, I learned that Regena had designed a technique for releasing old emotions that she called "swamping." She created it initially for herself. She was aware that her life was improving, but she was still struggling with depression and shame. The first time she "swamped," she listened to loud music, danced, stomped, and pounded pillows. She writes, "If we want to live healthy lives as women, we need the space to grieve our asses off as often as we feel moved."[71] Expressing our suppressed grief and rage and moving it through our bodies can be profoundly liberating.

At a retreat in Mexico with Regena and over 200 other women, all of us swamped together. Imagine getting in touch with what you think are your darkest feelings, with a couple hundred other women doing the same. I wanted to f-ing *run* out of that ballroom. Knowing the next hour would be very intense, I found a relatively quiet corner. I slowly began to do some of the movements Regena and her team had shared with us. I pushed against a wall, pushing and pushing and saying, "NOOO!" After some time passed, I started to experience surges of what felt like electricity going up my spine. The harder I pushed that wall and the more intense I felt about my NO, the more connected I felt to myself and my body. I was coming alive and letting go of old miseries—buried trauma.

I also twisted up a small white hotel towel and hit a table with it over and over and over. The sound the towel made as it hit the table and the movement of my arm gave me a sense of freedom in my body. My breath was deep. I was aware that my eyes were seeing the wall, the towel, and the table—more clearly. There was so much energy pulsating in my body. I had never allowed myself to be so wild and unbound. I had a few memories surface as I was swamping, but for the most part, my mind was still. I was just pushing that wall, whipping that towel, fully present. That night as I sat with some girlfriends on the beach under the stars, I remember feeling so very clear, powerful, and free, and the experience has continued to evolve.

Moving my energy in this way has helped me heal the trauma that was stored in my body, as well as release a deeper layer of being compliant and accommodating—essentially letting go of the limitations of being a "good girl." I had reclaimed not only more of my life-force energy but more of my sexual energy. I felt awake and turned on with life.

Two years after this retreat, I began to disentangle myself from my marriage. Both of us were very unhappy, and I was recognizing my role in our intense difficulties and uncovering more of my challenging patterns of codependency. With as much love as possible, I began the divorce process. Swamping is one of the many tools I used to reclaim myself and to feel fully alive.

Us

As we age, our sexuality changes. With the decline of hormones in our bodies, so many changes happen that can turn us off. Take, for example, one of the symptoms of menopause. Night sweats aren't sexy, and they disturb our sleep, which can affect our mental and emotional well-being. We can begin to feel betrayed by our bodies. In fact, in a recent survey, 83% of American women in menopause reported that they are dissatisfied with their bodies.[72] On the other hand, some studies show that sexual satisfaction increases with age. According to Jancee Dunn, more than half of sexually active women over the age of eighty report sexual "satisfaction" happens "almost always."[73] That's impressive—and we are assuming that these eighty-plus-year-old satisfied women know their way around their bodies and are probably vocal with their partners about their needs and desires. Please, let's not wait until we are eighty!

Being turned on is being connected to our spirit and life-force energy, believing in our ability and our power to create our lives, manifesting our desires, and *own our pussies*. Midlife or not, the more intense and demanding our lives are, the more we need to attend to what lights us up and evokes our pleasure.

Julie

And if you are uncomfortable with the word pussy ... so were we. *Very* uncomfortable. But now we love it. And most of our friends love it too! Pussies are strong as hell, and if you have any questions, see the Trevor Noah video in our book portal! What word did you use when you were younger? What word do you use now? Yoni, pee-pee, VJJ, taco, my privates, my poochie coochie, velvet glove, cooter, lady parts, hoo-ha, and finally, vagina (an inaccurate term, by the way). We reclaimed the word pussy. It belongs to us now, and our pussies do too! We suggest you do the same. We invite you to choose a word for yours that lights you up! I also use the word yoni because as a long-time meditator, I love the language of Sanskrit. Yoni translates to "sacred gateway."

ANATOMY OF EXTERNAL FEMALE GENETALIA

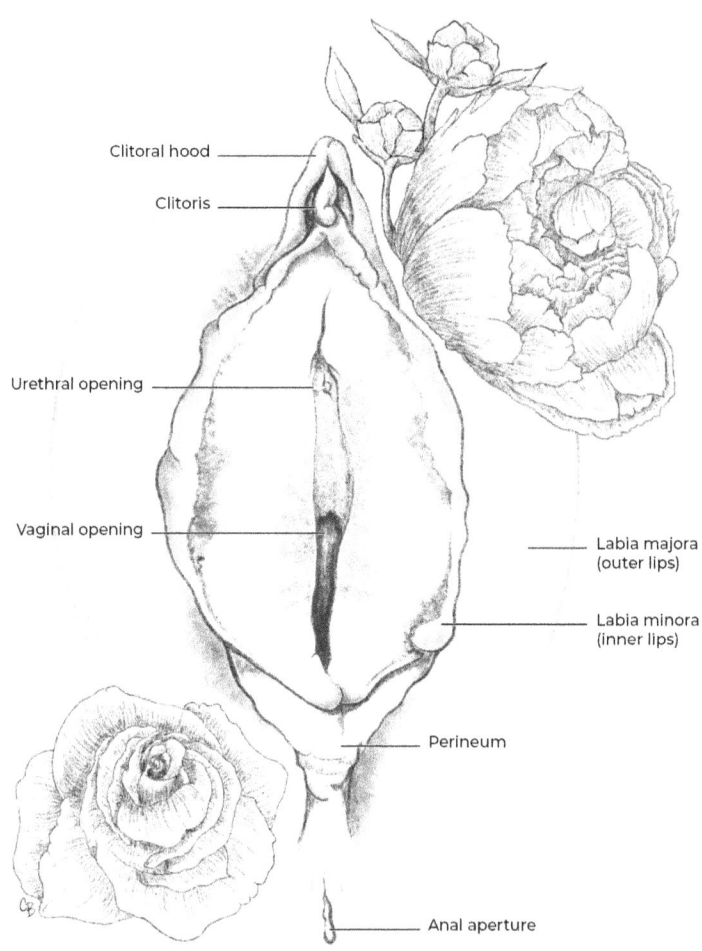

Sexuality advocate and educator Pamela Samuelson shares that "naming the female sex organ according to our preferences is of enormous importance, simply because naming it asserts our unique connection to and our power over our bodies."[74] Truth.

Some pussy education: Our pussy is more than just our vagina. "Vagina" is a Latin word meaning sheath. We don't know about you, but we are nobody's sheath! The vagina is a three-to-six-inch-long muscular canal from the cervix (the lowest part of the uterus) to the outside of the body. The vulva includes all of it—the labia, clitoris, and vaginal opening.

ANATOMY OF THE CLITORIS

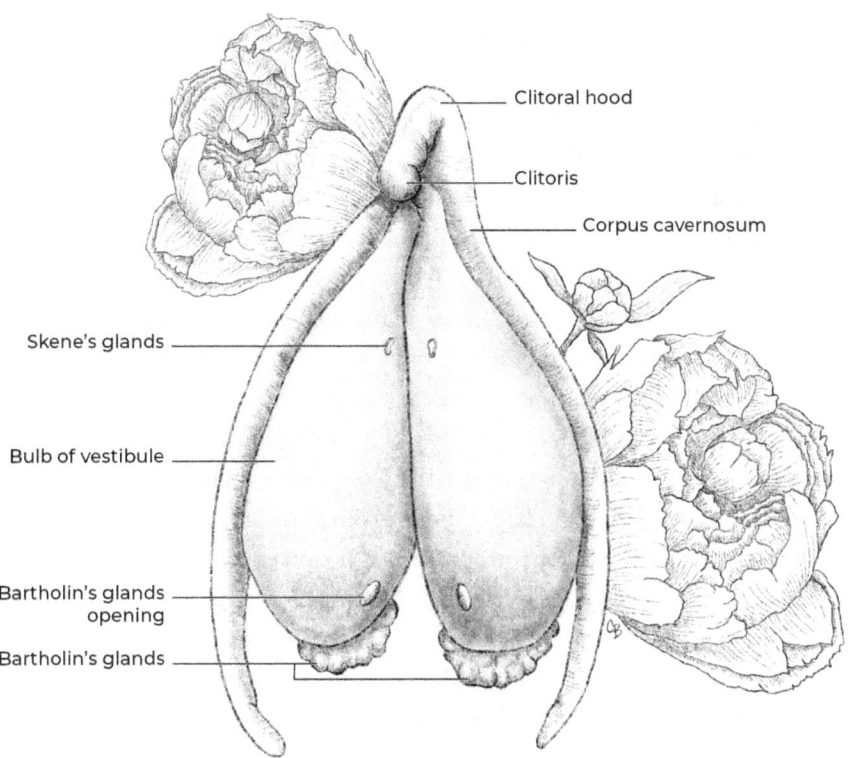

Bartholin's Glands: Produce and secrete mucous to aid in vaginal lubrication.

Skene's Glands: Produce and secrete substances that lubricate the opening of the urethra. The secreted substance is thought to be antimicrobial in efforts to prevent urinary tract infections. The Skene's glands also swell during sexual arousal.

Bulb of Vestibule: During sexual arousal, the bulb of vestibule becomes engorged with blood. This puts pressure on the corpus cavernosum and clitoris which creates a pleasant feeling during arousal.

Reference: Nguyen, J., D., &Duong, H. (2003) Anatomy, abdomen, and pelvis: Female external genitalia. National Library of Medicine.

Julie

Let's make some discoveries about our anatomy. I didn't take a really good look at my pussy until around five years ago... I was fifty-five years old. About eighteen years earlier, I had a beautiful baby, but not once did I check myself out. Wasn't that the job of the doctor and the midwife? Now I see what a disempowering strategy that was. I did have the good sense to fire my first OB/GYN when I told her I might squat during labor, and her response was, "I'm not going to get on the floor and deliver a baby." I thought I was the one delivering the baby, and her job was to support me! It wasn't until I was full-on menopausal that I used a mirror to make sure everything was looking good.

Because I have only been sexual with men, it had never dawned on me that a woman's genitalia might look different than mine. I assumed they all kinda looked the same. Seems like a crazy assumption now. They do not. They are each unique. Like a fingerprint or the lines on your palm. All pussies are flawless. And I haven't researched it (yet!), but I have a feeling that the unique appearance of each woman's pussy is a reflection of her personality, of her very soul.

Now let's take a big leap. Even if you have previously done some gazing at your lovely pussy, we suggest that you get a hand mirror and take a longer look. It's never too late to honor your extraordinary female anatomy. And if you desire for your partner to honor, enjoy, and respect your pussy, worshipping yourself helps the fulfillment of that desire.

You can do this in a very matter-of-fact way and do a little "inspection." That's fine, and it may be a good place to start. I started on my bathroom floor with a mirror scooched up between my legs, my reading glasses on, trying to get a good look. But we would invite you to create a sacred space by lighting a candle, choosing some lovely music, lying comfortably on your bed or a soft blanket, using some coconut oil for a massage, and offering her flowers, a gentle touch, and reverent viewing. Imagine you are giving your very best friend the most amazing gift imaginable. Our genitalia love to be honored and cherished. She has been in the dark for way too long.

If you are feeling like no f-ing way am I doing this—ever! Listen to this amazing podcast with Mel Robbins and sexpert Dr. Emily Morse. Mel was definitely NOT joining the pussy gazing posse. But Emily changed her mind. To listen, click on the QR Code in the beginning or the end of our book.

If you would like to take your pussy gazing further, yoni self-massage can awaken your libido and gently help you make a connection with a part of yourself that may be unfamiliar. Make sure your hands are warm, have your natural lubrication of choice nearby, and look at the illustrations of the anatomy of your vulva and clitoris. Simply begin to touch yourself.

Notice what feels good as well as where there might be tension or pain. Explore your own body and breathe. It helps to breathe slowly and deeply, at least four counts in and four counts out. Rhythmic breathing will support you in making a stronger connection to your body. And *very* important for us vulva owners: Women need an average of six to twenty minutes of arousal to experience an orgasm.[75] Take your time. If you are feeling uncomfortable emotions, allow yourself to experience them. Let go of any discomfort that you may be holding in your body.

Awakening our pussies has supported us in awakening so many other aspects of our lives. If you would like to learn more, there are quite a few, wonderful online courses taught by amazing women who can support you.

Let's talk some more about our pleasure. When we Googled "how many nerve endings on . . ." the first word that came up for us was "foreskin." Clitoris was a bit further down in our search. Prior research done on the female clitoris came from studying . . . wait for it . . . a cow. That study determined there are 8,000 nerve endings in a cow clitoris. In 2022, scientists finally decided to examine a woman and learned there are over 10,000 nerve endings in the human clitoris.[76]

Women are built for pleasure and orgasm. It's all about our pleasure! We have a short "refractory period," which simply means that we can enjoy multiple orgasms. The refractory period for men is much longer, and therefore, they need a longer recovery time between orgasms. And the penis is not exclusively for pleasure. It is multifunctional; it can urinate, ejaculate, and experience pleasure. The clitoris, however, exists *solely* for pleasure. That is *not* an anatomical error. And perhaps it is also not surprising to learn that the clitoris has been largely ignored by medical science. (Remember the cow?) Medical textbooks being published today continue to have many pages of anatomical pictures of the penis, while the clitoris and vulvar anatomy receive limited mention.

Urologist Helen O'Connell was the first to map the full anatomy and nerve pathways of the clitoris. Her first study was in 1998 (!), and she did a subsequent study in 2005 that examined the clitoris with an MRI. She discovered that it was a nerve-rich glans that extended beneath the pubic bone and wrapped around the vaginal opening and had bulbs that, when aroused, become engorged. Current medical curricula and research continue to disregard information about clitoral anatomy and function. O'Connell has shared, "We see (medical) literature doubting the importance of female orgasm, entertaining the argument that from an evolutionary standpoint, female orgasm could merely be a by-product of selection on male orgasm."[77] Remember the movie *When Harry Met Sally* and the fabulous orgasm in the deli? We are sure Sally Albright (played by Meg Ryan) would beg to differ on that one.

Additionally, the G-spot is part of the clitoral root that extends into the vagina. G-spot orgasms seem mythical for some women—the stuff of legend. We simply don't talk about it with each other enough. So, over the past few years, we have been discussing sexuality with our clients and friends, asking questions about G-spot, cervical orgasms, and ejaculation. Yes, that's right, female vaginal ejaculation. According to the data, most women only experience clitoral orgasms. By doing some research and taking online classes, we discovered there may be a whole world of pleasure that we are missing. The ability to orgasm, have the seemingly unattainable G-spot and cervical orgasms, plus ejaculate, are learnable skills. This isn't just about our sexuality; it's about being turned on with life, having confidence, being comfortable in our skin, and knowing **we deserve pleasure.**

And if you need further confirmation of the power of prioritizing our pleasure, here is some scientific data: "Orgasm and arousal release biochemicals like adrenaline and dopamine, which stimulate awareness, cognitive functioning, and mood. It also releases oxytocin, the so-called love hormone that can help partners feel bonded and even enhance relationship satisfaction," according to Dr. Brooke Faught, DNP.[78] It also protects against heart disease by raising your heart rate and lowering blood pressure, boosts the immune system, and can even support a better night's sleep.

Pam

I grew up in a conservative, midwestern town with conservative parents. Sex was not something that was discussed. At all. So I am not sure why or how, but I have always been a sexual person; I just didn't know it until I was in college. I somehow discovered. . . the vibrator. And life would never be the same. I thought to myself, "Why doesn't every woman know about these? And why don't they sell batteries in 100 packs?!"

I tended to be pretty open with my friends about sex. I mean, who doesn't want to know about what feels good? I made it my mission to tell all my close friends about vibrators, and if you didn't have one, there is a good chance I may have gifted you one or dragged you to the store to buy one. You know who you are.

As I got older and traveled more, I began to see how open the Europeans are about sex and how stuffy we are in the United States. It's a bit of a tragedy really—and something I've learned most women are curious about, but we just don't talk about it.

Us

Our beautiful vulvas have meridians and reflexology zones. Different parts correspond to the different glands and organs of our bodies. Awakening our bodies by caring for and nourishing our vulvas is deeply healing. In the past few years, there have been many wonderful products introduced, particularly for midlife women, that support and nourish our labia and vagina, as well as some CBD products that encourage arousal and lubrication. There is even a product, Vella Women's Pleasure Serum, that helps with arousal, sensation, and enhanced orgasm. Carolyn Wheeler, co-founder of Vella, says, "Vella ushers in a whole new era of agency over our bodies. We can better claim our right to pleasure. And, as we see it, pleasure is power."[79] Well, it is about time! Pleasure IS power. Now, if insurance companies would cover and honor women's pleasure, too, that would be real progress! (Erectile dysfunction meds are basically free!) Many of the companies that have emerged in this FemTech space are founded by women, approaching women's sexual health very differently in an industry (tech) dominated by men. Glorious.

For many women in midlife, after choosing to end long and unfulfilling relationships or marriages, a more delightful and fulfilling sex life comes roaring back. Others have chosen to focus on upgrading their current relationships and sexuality. Others are having the time of their life, enjoying the company of friends, and maybe dating. It doesn't have to be a traditional relationship; you just have to be open to the possibilities of your desires. We have quite a few midlife friends who have shared with us that they had no idea that their sex life could be so incredibly *goooood*. In midlife, we may now finally have the opportunity to focus on ourselves, because we are no longer beholden to the needs and desires of our partners, children, or our society.

Our friends and clients have shared some amazing words offered by their now attentive partners: "Your pussy is magic!" "My pleasure is pleasuring you." "You are so delicious." And you do not have to wait for a partner to admire and honor you. Sex therapist and author of *Smart Sex*, Dr. Emily Morse, shares that we should begin our day with a "Meditate, Masturbate, Manifest" morning routine. "Meditation is an important practice to clear my thoughts. Masturbation allows me to connect to my body and ground in pleasure. Manifestation channels my vision for the day."[80] It is wonderful and essential to love and adore ourselves.

We know a lovely woman, Diana, who has struggled with her sexuality. She was sexually abused as a child and, as a result, lacked real intimacy in her past relationships. Diana had multiple failed marriages and, at age fifty-three, was about ready to just accept that she should be single forever. Fortunately, Diana found an amazing therapist who not only helped her unpack her trauma but also recommended that she see a sex therapist. Reluctantly, Diana saw the sex therapist and learned something very interesting about herself: She was a deeply sexual person, but the abuse and shame had made her deny those parts of herself.

Diana decided to start dating again but wasn't finding what she wanted. We encouraged her to make a desire list. To sit down, meditate, and write down what she truly desired in a man and what would bring her pleasure. What kept coming to her was that she wanted a lover—a man who would be there just to satisfy her sexually with no expectations of a big relationship. She found her man almost instantly, a hot, younger man! She says they have a friendship and intimacy on a different level since there are no expectations of a long-term commitment. The sex is amazing, and Diana says that in her fifties, she is discovering things about herself she never knew. For the first time in her life, Diana feels like she has complete control over her mind, emotions, body, and sexuality. Having agency has given Diana an energy we haven't seen in her before—she is glowing.

In a 2021 interview with *The Guardian*, artist Marina Abramovic shared that "Many people think after menopause, women give up the idea of sex. For me, sex since then has never been better, because you don't have to worry about pregnancy. Right now, I have a boyfriend who is twenty-one years younger. I see sex as a necessary balance, along with good food, humor, joy for life."[81]

We love going on and on about the importance of female pleasure; however, if there are any symptoms of menopause affecting your lady parts, the idea of pleasure may seem unattainable. Some of the symptoms that can affect our sexuality are pelvic-floor issues, frequent urinary tract infections, vaginal dryness, vaginal atrophy, difficulty with orgasm, and reduced libido. Just typing this list bums us out. 44% of women experience some kind of sexual dysfunction, but most women *do not* report theirs to their physician, and most doctors don't ask.[82] Maybe many of us use the "grin and bear it" method, just hoping our symptoms—and our sex lives—will get better. Or we are uncomfortable talking about it and asking, "I would like to have a healthy sex life. Can you share some suggestions that can support me during menopause?" There are many actions we can take that will help us enjoy our sexuality and maintain a happy and healthy life.

We are lucky to know some outstanding female practitioners who are very knowledgeable about perimenopause, menopause, and much more. You may want to seek out a provider that specializes in menopause, women's sexual health, and female urology. We will be honest here: Neither of us would be completely comfortable discussing our sex lives with a male practitioner. Sorry. And, of course, as mentioned in an earlier chapter, medical schools offer very little training in perimenopausal or menopausal care, and OB/GYNs may dismiss the issues entirely. However, since menopause has recently become such a hot topic, more doctors are pursuing continuing education in the field of women's health and, specifically, menopause. You just have to ask the questions! And when in doubt, ask your girlfriends.

In one study by the Women's Nutritional Advisory Service, "nearly 40% of menopausal women are being prescribed antidepressants to help manage their symptoms, despite 4 out of 5 of those women describing that antidepressant treatment was 'inappropriate.'"[83] It also is worth mentioning that challenging sexual side effects are known to be very common with antidepressants. Many years ago, during early perimenopause, both of us were seeing highly recommended male practitioners who prescribed antidepressants for us, never asking any questions regarding our perimenopausal symptoms.

We have to advocate for ourselves. And maybe take a girlfriend or loving sister with you to your appointment so she can support you with feeling comfier and taking notes!

Questions to Ask Your Practitioner:

- Sex can be very painful, and I don't seem to be lubricating like I used to. Do you have recommendations?
- My libido seems to be disappearing. My orgasms don't seem as enjoyable. They are different than they used to be. What are your suggestions?
- Would talking to a sex therapist be helpful for me? Do you have someone you trust and would recommend?
- I've heard that hormone therapy might help increase my libido. Do you have any experience with this? Are there supplements or natural approaches to consider as well?
- I have recently developed some anxiety regarding sex. I pretend to be asleep when my partner tries to initiate sex. What is happening?
- Would blood tests be useful to determine what is going on with my hormones and sex drive?

Julie

A couple of years ago, I developed a UTI (urinary tract infection) for the first time in my life. I made an emergency appointment with my beloved female physician. During my exam, she told me that I had vaginal atrophy. Um, what the hell is vaginal atrophy? Well, now that I am sixty, my vaginal walls are thinning. It's the "if you don't use it, you lose it" effect, just like with muscles.

So I took immediate action and began doing vaginal exercises using a jade egg. (Don't knock the jade egg just because a famous Goop gal got in trouble for promoting its benefits.) "By fortifying your pelvic floor, yoni eggs can amplify your intimate experiences, boost the number and quality of orgasms, and improve overall pelvic health."[84] Doing vaginal exercises with a jade egg is similar to doing Kegel exercises.[85] And Kegels were *always* intended to be done with weights in the vagina. Repeat that for the ladies in the back! Otherwise, it's like you are flapping your vaginal walls around with nothing to push against. If you want a strong vagina, you need resistance training! And believe me—a strong vagina is a happy pussy. In our book portal, we recommend wonderful businesses, some female-owned, that offer products that will support your sexual health.

Formerly known as vaginal atrophy and renamed in 2014, Genitourinary Syndrome of Menopause (GSM) refers to the symptoms that can occur to the vulva-vaginal-urinary system. These symptoms can be very painful, are dangerous for our long-term health, and affect over 50-70% of women.[86] GSM can occur during perimenopause, worsen with menopause, and is a condition that manifests when the ovaries produce less estrogen. There will be a thinning, drying, and inflammation of the vaginal walls that can lead to distressing urinary symptoms and more. Even walking, wearing pants, and wiping with toilet paper can cause agony for some women. GSM remains extremely underdiagnosed despite being a serious health challenge and rarely resolves if left untreated. Please take a deep breath before you read this list.

SOME OF THE GSM SIGNS AND SYMPTOMS

- Vaginal dryness, burning, itching
- Genital itching
- Frequency, urgency, and burning with urination
- Incontinence
- Recurrent urinary tract infections
- Pain during intercourse
- Bleeding after intercourse
- Decreased vaginal lubrication

- Shortening and tightening of the vaginal canal

- And a symptom that is rarely shared: atrophy (let us be clear—shrinking) of the inner and outer labia

Our clients and friends who have GSM have shared with us that oral or penetrative sex can become *very* painful. Orgasming becomes more difficult. UTIs become frequent. We are losing vulvar, clitoral and vaginal sensation and integrity. All of this turns women off to sex. And just for confirmation here: The Menopause Society has reported that 45% of menopausal women experience pain during sex.[87] That means if you are meeting two of your girlfriends for lunch, the odds are that one of them may be suffering silently. Have the conversation—talk about sex! There are gentle solutions, and we need to share the good news.

Vaginal estrogen cream, suppositories, and rings can be beneficial for preventing UTIs and can help restore vaginal tissue so they're less dry, and therefore, sex will be more pleasurable, too. A 2014 review of forty-four studies found that vaginal estrogen resolved ALL of GSM's major symptoms.[88] Dr. Rachel Rubin, a board-certified urologist and sexual medicine specialist, has shared, "Genitals are very hormone-sensitive and hormone-dependent structures. Without supple tissue, female sex organs become dry and thin. Arousal becomes physically difficult and intercourse can be agonizing. Unfortunately, the medical community doesn't spend a lot of time on these topics. Women shouldn't be waking up multiple times a night to urinate. They shouldn't be getting recurring infections."[89]

Rubin believes that every woman, during her annual physical when she turns forty-five, should receive a prescription for local vaginal estrogen! Vaginal estrogen reduces the chance of recurrent UTIs by 50-75%.[90] There is quite a buzz about this as more women are demanding vaginal estrogen for their long-term health—and to improve their sex lives. More physicians are getting on board.

Dr. Kelly Casperson has said that vaginal estrogen therapy should be lifelong *and* inexpensive. She has said, "I want to see $4 vaginal cream at Walmart. I'm manifesting that into the universe."[91] Unfortunately, for now, these treatments can be quite costly. Estrogen treatment for our genitals is very low-dose, and according to Casperson, a year's worth of vaginal estrogen is equivalent to taking one low-dose pill of estrogen HT (hormone therapy). Make sure you are using it according to the prescribed instructions. Even too much of a good thing can have systemic consequences. Vaginal estrogen is readily available through many online healthcare providers, too. We have some clients who use prescription DHEA cream vaginally (a precursor to estrogen and testosterone) instead of estrogen, and this has offered them some relief from dryness, painful burning, and sexual discomfort.

We love this comment by the powerhouse Dr. Somi Javaid, Founder of HerMD in an email: "We remember moisturizer for our face, hands, and feet. But a lot of women forget about moisturizing sensitive parts like the vagina and vulva."[92] Taking good care of your yoni during midlife is essential, even if your symptoms are minimal. Using softer toilet tissue or biodegradable wipes (especially if you are prone to UTIs) and urinating after sexual activity can be very helpful.

There are also pain-free vaginal laser treatments to strengthen and thicken the vaginal walls. The Kegel throne is supposed to be very effective, too. You can sit on what looks like a chair and experience 11,000 kegels per minute. And a side benefit—it is supposed to feel gooood. We haven't tried this, so we don't know if it's effective or if the results are lasting, but we mention it to illustrate the range of possibilities. If you aren't into the jade egg and thrones, there are other amazing devices, from crystal wands to silicone vibrators, that help you do self-healing from the comfort of your own home to develop a beautiful, powerful, and very healthy pussy for as long as you both shall live!

BENEFITS OF INTIMACY, SEX, AND ORGASMS IN MIDLIFE (EVEN IF IT'S WITH YOURSELF!)

- Keeps you young by improving circulation
- Promotes release of endorphins
- Stress reliever: reduces your cortisol levels

- Releases oxytocin, a mood lifter
- Improves your sleep and sleep quality
- Better relationship with partner if you have one—if not, better relationship with yourself!
- Strengthens your pelvic floor muscles
- Helps relieve body aches
- Immune-system booster
- Supports confidence and self-esteem

Pussify It!

Another way to delight yourself and bring more pleasure into your life is to pussify it! (Gratitude to Regena Thomashauer for debuting "pussify" into our lexicon!) Let's consider a reinvention of Marie Kondo's brilliant concept of keeping only those things that spark joy in our lives. Though we are almost certain that she'd never use the word pussify, what if there were a cleaning and sorting process where we chose to surround ourselves with the things that spark joy for our pussies?! You can create more space for more beauty and MORE of your desires. Adorn yourself with clothes that feel good on your body. Perhaps create a space in your home that is *exclusively* yours—maybe you could repurpose a corner of your bedroom. How about those closets, boxes in your basement (that's a metaphor for sure!), and even your friends of many years that you have outgrown? Pussify them! Do old sheets on your bed bring you joy and light you up? Time for new sheets! Want a super delicious upgrade? Buy yourself some sexy lingerie. Or warm slippers. Whatever turns *you* on—just for *your* pleasure. Treat yourself to pleasures and desires as you would a dear friend . . . or amp it up, give it your all, and be your own hottest lover.

Kasia Urbaniak spent seventeen years studying to become a Taoist nun while working as one of the most successful dominatrixes in the world. Read that sentence again and let yourself experience the visuals!

Her income from being a dominatrix paid for her studies with the nuns. (By the way, being a dominatrix does not include sex.) She authored the book *Unbound: A Woman's Guide to Power*. In her book and classes, she shares a simple yet very provocative exercise asking women to create a desire list. She writes, "True desires are a message from you to you, about what will make you feel truly alive. Because knowing what feeds you, what lights you up, and what you can plug into that will always nourish and inspire you, is the power of desire. Knowing what we want is a prerequisite for moving powerfully through the world."[93]

Take a moment now to create your desire list. Get out your journal or your phone. We encourage you to imagine this list filled with wild dreams that delight you, lift your heart, and even feel sensational to your pussy. No desire is too outrageous. We may not permit ourselves, nor does our culture, to feel our lustiest desires, earth-shattering as well as simple. We may spend much of our lives trying to hold it all together. As Kasia says, "Maybe what you are imagining is wild, generative, and hilarious; maybe it would blow up your life. Both are great." And don't bother with the cursed "hows"—this list is not about *how* it will happen. Just let your desires flow, flow, flow. Give this gift to yourself now. Begin designing your delicious desires and your life. I desire...

PAM

I desire ridiculous abundance—financial, health, spirit, and in friendships! I desire to uplift and support all women because our world needs more powerful women to step up, now more than ever. I desire to take my supportive and loving husband on a wonderful vacation to Sicily for some beautiful sunshine, swimming in the Ionian Sea, and amazing Italian food. I imagine us in a luxurious hotel room, falling asleep to the smells and sounds of the sea.

JULIE

I desire that all women everywhere have access to clean water, healthy food, safe homes, and education. That they are free from abuse and violence and have the support of their communities to create more peace and happiness in our world. I desire to be deliciously abundant, to spend time in one of my favorite places in the world, New York City, and to be a happy and generous mother and grandmother. I desire that my "late love" and I have a soulful and deeply loving relationship that elevates my entire life. And that we have an enormous amount of eros (and great sex) for all of our lives together.

Now, let's do a mini-meditation. **To listen along, click on the QR Code at the beginning or the end of our book.** Take a look at your desires, then gently close your eyes. Breathe in deeply. Breathe out long. Breathe into your heart. Breathe out from your heart. Now, breathe into your lower belly. And breathe out from your lower belly. Let's bring some of those desires into your future reality. Imagine yourself three years from now. Imagine that your wildest desires have come true.

- How are you feeling in your body? What sensations are you experiencing?
- What does your life look like? What is different?
- How have your desires changed your life?
- What have you let go of?
- How have you upgraded your life?
- Who are you spending time with?
- Do you have even more SECRET desires sparkling in your heart?

And now, say to yourself: "And so shall it be, or something even more amazing!" You can choose to write about your longings and desires so you can enjoy and reference them later. You might even want to create a vision board representing your beautiful desires.

Some Questions to Contemplate:

- Where do you enjoy being touched?
- Is there any place on your body that is off limits?
- What is one of your biggest turn-ons?
- How do you like being kissed?
- Which area of your body do you consider the sexiest?
- Are there words that would turn you on?
- Do you have some sexual fantasies?
- How frequently would you enjoy having sex?
- Are there some things that might be taboo during love-making?

Midlife is a time to discover more about what turns you on. It means taking the time to love and nourish yourself, letting go of disapproval and shame, choosing to define sexuality on *your* terms, and beginning to focus on what *you* desire and what pleases *you*. Your pleasure originates with you and belongs to you. Sex in the second half of life can be the best!

Reclaiming your sexuality at midlife is a profoundly personal exploration and can be a passage to a life filled with more love, pleasure, and enjoyment. This is the time to reclaim more of our life force and power! No more worries about pregnancy or periods, so let's enjoy our sexuality. If not now, then when? All women deserve a Midlife Upgrade. As the brilliant urologist Dr. Casperson writes in *You Are Not Broken*, "I love myself enough to have a happy sex life."[94]

CHAPTER 5

SELF-CARE IS THE NEW SELF-CARE

"Almost everything will work again if you unplug it for a few minutes, including you."
—Anne Lamott

"Self-care is giving the world the best of you, instead of what's left of you."
—Katie Reed

Hold on to your hot flashes because we are going to talk about some basics here: Self. Care. Why are women tired? All. The. Time. The stage of life when menopause tends to happen can be particularly demanding. Here you are, navigating the menopausal maze where leggings are your best friend. You don't even remember the last time you had a good night's sleep, and lurking in the shadows is the neglect gremlin. He's got you managing parents, kids, the family schedule, your job, and the household. He loves it when you are constantly people-pleasing, scrolling social media, and saying yes to everything and no to yourself. He's cleverly disguised as perfection, self-sacrifice, guilt, comparison, business, chocolate, a caffeine fix, and wine.

We want to be clear—there can be a lot of "fake" self-care out there:

serums, body scrubs, candles, bubble baths, weighted blankets, LED face masks, "retail therapy," even indulging in endless self-help books and programs. Interestingly enough, many of these items are marketed exclusively to women, and while these things may be luxuriously indulgent, they are not always true self-care. Why should we need to run out and buy things for our outside when we just need to take care of our inside?

Here's the deal, dearest: Self-care is self-love. It means taking care of your physical, emotional, and mental well-being. Self-care is not a quick, temporary fix, but is essential for maintaining a healthy and balanced life—so a bubble bath is a true luxury and not just an escape from your everyday life. The onset of menopause can be exhausting mentally, physically, and emotionally, so if you have been neglecting yourself up until now, it's time to honor the magnificent woman you are!

We have coached a lot of women who put themselves last. Women today are told they can be superwomen. You can have it all! Work a full-time job! Raise a family! Be the cook, chauffeur, and housekeeper! Entertain and be social! Work out! But at what cost? Think about it. Even if you wake up after suffering from a night of restless sleep and night sweats, you will still get up and have things to do: feed and let the dog out, get to that important meeting, or take care of your children's needs (while your partner is snoring next to you). Too often, women will choose to care for the needs of others over their own. This is especially true for women who are caregivers for children, elderly parents, or other family members, which many midlife women are.

You are already doing some forms of self-care as habits you may not consciously recognize as being self-care practices. Count these as self-care wins!

- **Personal grooming:** Shower, brush your teeth, and dress in a way that makes you feel good.

- **Taking breaks:** Either step away from work or give yourself some downtime.

- **Hobbies:** Reading, cooking, and crafting provide pleasure and relaxation.

- **Spending time in nature:** Whether it's a walk or bike ride, many people naturally gravitate to spending time outside.
- **Socializing:** Spend time with loved ones or just enjoy someone else's company.
- **Listen to music** or do creative activities like dancing and singing.

Now that you are aware you already have some self-care wins, you might be able to expand on those to incorporate new habits into your life. We are going to give you tips on how to do that. Self-care, like any other discipline, involves setting goals, establishing routines, and practicing good habits that promote overall wellness and rejuvenation. It means making choices that prioritize *you* even when you face demands or distractions. We all want to be fabulously healthy, have tons of energy, and enjoy a long, happy life. But only you hold the key to achieving those things—it's right inside you. You alone hold the power to create your happiness.

Why is it that we aren't first on the list? Well, there are several reasons you may not even be aware of. Even though we are in the twenty-first century, we are still unfortunately living in a patriarchal society where expectations of men and women are different (anybody here see the Barbie movie? That monologue said it all!). Our cultural and societal norms are that women should prioritize the needs of others over themselves. Think about it. If the kids are dirty, no one says to the dad, "Hey, your kid is dirty." If the house is messy, no one blames the man for not cleaning up. Those expectations are almost always placed on the woman or mother. We feel obligated. We feel judged. Ugh. Good old patriarchal double standards.

Many women tend to feel guilty or ashamed for prioritizing themselves over others. Today's women are juggling many responsibilities like work, childcare, household duties, caring for aging parents, and social engagements—which leaves them with little time for themselves. Often, women lack the support they need to prioritize themselves, whether it be help with childcare, financial support, or even emotional support. To top it all off, society places a lot of pressure on women to be and look a certain way, and that can lead to feelings of low self-esteem and low self-worth.

Our modern world is also one that glorifies business and productivity. But if you're here, we bet you already know that. We truly believe this is one of the reasons why midlife women are so tired. Well, that and the constant night-waking and night sweats. Taking the time to tend to oneself is more important now than ever. As health and life coaches, we have worked with many women who want to know about what foods to eat and how to nourish their bodies. We are here to tell you that you can eat all the healthy foods you want, but if you don't tend to yourself, you will feel depleted. When you take the time to nurture your mind, body, and spirit, you are able to show up as your authentic self, live life to its fullest, and have more to give to others.

We have already discussed the importance of drinking water and eating a healthy diet, which is certainly important, but there are some other things you might consider working into your life so that you are the best version of yourself. You are worthy of love, compassion, and care.

Here's the deal: Menopause is *real*. And it can last for years. If you are dealing with difficulties from sleep issues to sweating to mood changes to low libido to just feeling yucky in general, now is the time more than ever to put yourself first. Self-care during the menopausal years is a way to recognize this transition as well as a way to honor and nurture this profound life change.

If you need ways to better practice self-care, here are some things to consider: Say no. That's right. We are permitting you to say *no*. Learning to say no can be one of the most important tools in your self-care kit because it helps you set boundaries and prioritize your own needs. By the way, saying no isn't selfish or rude, so don't feel guilty about taking time to make space for what matters to you. When you learn to say no, you are showing yourself and others that your time and energy are valuable. If this is something you struggle with, here are some ways to politely say no:

- "No, sorry, I cannot do that."
- "I appreciate your kind offer, but I must decline."

- "I wish I could, but I have other commitments."
- "I'm sorry, but I won't be able to help you out this time."
- "Thanks for thinking of me, but I'm going to have to pass."
- "I would love to, but if I don't get some rest, I'm going to take a hostage."

See—it's not that hard!

How Do You Know When to Say No?

- You are already over-scheduled.
- The event doesn't vibe with your values or goals.
- It might negatively impact your mental or physical health.
- You are agreeing to do something to avoid guilt (out of obligation or fear of disappointing others).
- You are already dreading the event.
- Your intuition is telling you no!

Saying no is one of the best things you can do to start serving yourself and creating boundaries. This is one of the things that is at the heart of self-care. You cannot pour from an empty cup.

We once coached a lovely woman, Sarah, who was exhausted all the time. She came to us looking for ways to modify her diet so that she would have more energy. When we dug in deeper, we learned Sarah not only managed her own four kids but was helping to raise her brother's son, running her household, caring for her aging parents, entertaining her husband's clients at dinner parties, on the board of her kids' PTA, volunteering at school, working out, doing her socializing with friends, and helping to fundraise for her church all while also holding down a full-time job. Unreal. Just hearing her to-do list would make anyone feel exhausted! Sarah was so used to doing everything for everyone that she didn't even notice how many things she was doing until we wrote it all down. Once we started to examine ways she could say no and hand tasks off to others, she almost immediately started to feel better—physically *and* mentally. Sarah finally began to prioritize herself. When found she had more patience with her family, was more productive at work, and was much happier and healthier!

Establish a Morning Routine and An Evening Routine (and Stick to Them!)

We have coached many women over the years and have found that morning and evening routines were the most important things to keeping their health on track. And here you thought routines were just for kids. Wrong! Routines are beneficial for so many reasons. They help reduce stress and anxiety by providing structure and predictability to your day. When you know what's coming, you'll feel less overwhelmed and more in control. When you have established routines, you'll likely stay more focused on your goals and feel more productive. Routines also help with building healthy habits, like scheduling time for exercise or meal planning. They are so good for overall mental and physical well-being.

Let's start with a morning routine. A good morning routine can set the tone for your day. It does not have to be complicated or time-consuming. And once established, it will become a habit. You may have to experiment to find what works best for you—but here are a few ideas to get you started.

MORNING ROUTINE

- **Wake up at the same time every day:** Even on the weekends. Contrary to popular belief, sleeping longer on weekends may not help you recoup the sleep you lost through the week. Sleep experts say consistency is best for healthy sleep.[95] If you miss out on sleep on the weekends, just get back to the routine. And a nap will be more beneficial than trying to sleep in.

- **Hydrate first thing in the morning:** Keep a glass of water by the bed and drink it when you first wake up. You might be surprised at how good this makes you feel! If you think about it, you have probably been dehydrated during the night. Drinking a glass of water will help you wake up.

- **Try some stretching exercises or some light yoga** to wake your body up and improve flexibility.

- **Meditate or practice mindfulness:** We are going to tell you—this one habit has been life-changing for many of our clients. We know many women who have struggled to meditate for years. The common complaint was not being able to turn off the monkey brain. For clients who are struggling to shut off their brains, we suggest finding a guided meditation app. There are many meditation apps, including everything from intention setting to having a positive day to helping you just wake up. We cannot recommend this enough. It does not have to be long or complicated. Just start with three to five minutes and work your way up from there. Meditation is such a beautiful way to start your day. Go to the QR code at the end of the book to view some meditation apps we suggest.

- **Open Your Heart:** Louise Hay, the fabulous author of *You Can Heal Your Life*, suggests saying "I love you" when you first look at yourself in the mirror in the morning. Then, ask yourself, "How can I serve you today?"

- **Plan your day:** It is always beneficial to take a few minutes to map out your day and prioritize your tasks. You will find you are more focused and organized and less stressed!

EVENING ROUTINE

Let's talk about the evening routine. We already discussed how sleep-deprived many women are. Your evening routine is just as important, if not more important, than your morning routine. If you are struggling with getting yourself to bed in the evening, we suggest reframing your idea of going to bed at the start of your next day. It may help you to avoid putting off shutting down for the night. Having a solid nighttime routine will help you de-stress from the day, promote relaxation, get you in a peaceful state, and set you up for a great night of much-needed restful sleep.

- **Have a consistent sleep schedule:** As mentioned earlier, consistency is one of the keys to a good night's rest. Once you get into a regular sleeping pattern, your body will become used to shutting down at a certain time.

- **Wind down before bed:** Hey, we get it. Sometimes it sounds like a good idea to binge-watch Netflix after a long day. But that's not going to help you get better sleep. Take an hour before bed and do some relaxing activities like reading, taking a warm bath or shower, meditating, or journaling. Activities like these will help calm your mind down for rest. According to the National Center for Biotechnology Information, not only do warm baths or showers help you fall asleep faster, but they also improve sleep quality and lower blood pressure.[96] The theory is that warm water stimulates blood flow to the hands and feet, therefore allowing body heat to escape more quickly.

- **Avoid stimulating activities:** Playing video games, working, or vigorous exercise at night can rev your brain (and body) up and make it more difficult to sleep. Save activities like these for the day, when you have more energy and brain power. If you want to exercise at night, try walking, stretching, or doing light yoga.

- **Step away from your devices:** This is a tough one for a lot of us, and it's easier said than done. Everyone seems to be married to their phones, computers, and even televisions. But even if it's just for a short period, creating digital boundaries will have positive effects on your overall well-being, not just your sleep. Using devices right before bed disrupts sleep because they emit blue light that suppresses sleep hormones. You are tricking your brain into thinking it's daytime. Also, while you might look forward to them, continuous exposure to notifications (emails, texts, and social media updates) can be stressful and further keep you from restful sleep. If you must be on your phone or computer at night, invest in some blue-light-blocking readers or blue-blocker glasses (yes, they are out there, and yes, we have some).

- **Limit alcohol and caffeine:** Sorry, ladies, that glass of wine isn't going to help you sleep better. While alcohol initially makes you feel drowsy, it is a stimulant, and it may wake you up in the middle of the night. Both caffeine and alcohol are not only sleep disruptors and stimulants, but they are also diuretics. It's not fun to wake in the night with a full bladder! Definitely avoid alcohol and caffeine before bedtime if you are having trouble sleeping. This is a big one. In general, alcohol use in midlife is discouraged. Sorry ladies, but if you want to sleep, lose weight, and feel your best, you should avoid alcohol for several reasons. According to the National Institutes of Health, alcohol is both a stimulant and depressant.[97] It initially slows down the central nervous system, and after a couple of glasses of wine, you may fall asleep faster. However, later in the night, as alcohol levels in your body drop, your brain kicks into overdrive! The alcohol disrupts your sleep architecture, and you might pay for it in the second half of the night by tossing and turning as your body speeds through the sleep cycles. So, besides the calories that contribute to midlife weight gain, alcohol can keep you awake and prevent deep REM sleep so that even if you think you have slept well, you won't wake up feeling rested. Also, consuming alcohol can create uncomfortable symptoms close to bedtime, as increased heart rate and adrenaline can affect sleep.

Pam

I have struggled with sleep issues, and I still do from time to time. Sometimes, I have problems falling or staying asleep. I have struggled with waking up at night and not being able to get back to sleep. It's no picnic walking around in a sleep coma, and I'm sure my family can tell you I'm no peach when I'm tired. Having a solid sleep routine has been a game changer for me, and I work on it with my coaching clients as well. For me, the big things that made a difference were getting my hormones balanced, managing my evening phone and TV time, and managing stress levels with yoga nidra meditations. I wind down at night with a calming herbal tea like lemon balm or chamomile. I take magnesium glycinate, magnesium L-threonate, or Natural Calm, all of which have been found to reduce symptoms of insomnia and anxiety. I occasionally use CBD to help sleep, and I don't watch the news. Instead, I read to wind down before bed.

Us

Get seven to nine hours of sleep. We cannot stress enough how important sleep is! Sleeping is as important as eating a good diet and exercising. It's the foundation of good health, and inadequate sleep can seriously impact your health and quality of life. According to the Sleep Foundation, most adults do not get enough sleep.[98] Statistics show more than one in three Americans get less than seven hours of sleep per night, and during perimenopause and menopause, it may be less than seven hours.[99] According to the National Institutes of Health, 50% of menopausal women say they experience insomnia.[100]

Inadequate sleep can lead to some serious health issues, such as hypertension, obesity, diabetes, heart disease, stroke, and chronic mental stress, so it's important to address. We were those women who struggled with sleep! It's no fun walking around perpetually exhausted.

Why does it get so much worse for women in midlife? One of the main causes of insomnia, especially during perimenopause, is night sweats and hot flashes. These sudden bursts of heat don't only make it difficult to get to sleep, but if they happen in the middle of the night, it can become difficult to return to sleep. Those pesky hormones can also cause anxiety and depression, mood changes, and a change in lifestyle and routine, which can also lead to sleep disorders or insomnia. Perimenopause can also affect the circadian rhythm, which is the body's natural sleep-wake cycle. Hormone changes can make it difficult to fall asleep at night and wake up in the morning.

While most people think sleep is when the body completely shuts down, this is simply not true. It is the time your body needs to heal and recover, restore energy, repair cells, and release essential hormones.

GOOD SLEEP IS CRITICAL

- The body repairs and rejuvenates itself, cells regenerate, and the immune system strengthens.

- Sleep is so important for brain function, including memory consolidation, learning, problem-solving, and creativity. Lack of sleep can impair cognitive function, which makes it difficult to focus, concentrate, and make decisions.

- Sleep helps regulate the hormones that control metabolism, hunger, and stress. This is why you may crave sweets when you are tired! Lack of these hormones can lead to weight gain, insulin resistance, and increased risk for chronic disease.

- Mood boost! A good night's rest is essential for emotional well-being and most definitely impacts mood. Sleep deprivation can contribute to irritability, anxiety, and depression.

- Sleep also improves physical performance and is important for physical recovery—it's when your cells are rejuvenating!

TIPS FOR BETTER SLEEP

- **Make time for exercise during the day:** We all know exercise is important for overall health, and regular exercise also helps promote rest in the evening. Just don't exercise too close to bedtime, as increased heart rate and adrenaline can affect sleep.

- **Darken your bedroom:** You are more likely to fall asleep if your room is completely dark. You can also try wearing a sleep mask.

- **Meditate:** Yoga Nidra is a wonderful meditation that helps with sleep. We recommend Insight Timer to many of our coaching clients for sleep meditations. Listen to music or white noise—this can help you to relax and drown out any outside noises. YouTube has sleep music, like binaural beats and sleep meditations that can help with relaxation and sleep. You can get a sleep mask with headphones and listen while you fall asleep.

- **Read a book:** Reading is a great, low-key activity to help your brain wind down after a long day. Or —write in a journal. Journaling before bed is not only great for mental health, but it may also help you ease your mind before rest. Writing down your thoughts can help you process your day so you're not overthinking at night. You might even make your list of things to do for the next day so you don't ruminate during precious sleep time.

While no supplements will replace a good sleep routine, these are supplements that may help you get quality sleep:

- **Lemon balm** is a very calming herb. You can get it as a tea or a tincture and add a little honey, which helps your body release melatonin.

- **Melatonin** is a naturally occurring hormone your brain produces as a response to darkness. (Yet another reason to mind your screen time before bed.) While melatonin won't put you to sleep, it does help put you in a quiet state of relaxation. You don't need very much, only three milligrams, and more doesn't mean better.

- **Valerian** is an herb that can help you fall asleep faster and improve the quantity and quality of your sleep. There was an interesting study done in 2011 by the National Institutes of Health that showed a statistically significant change in the quality of sleep for women aged fifty to sixty who had been experiencing insomnia.[101] Added bonus: It may also help with hot flashes! Valerian does take some time to work, though, somewhere between two and four weeks.

- **Magnesium glycinate, magnesium bisglycinate or Magnesium Threonate:** Taking two hundred to five hundred milligrams around thirty minutes before bed can help with sleep. Magnesium is believed to help regulate neurotransmitters that are directly related to sleep. Like with melatonin, more may not be better; see what works for you.

- **L-theanine** is a commonly derived amino acid that promotes relaxing brain activity. This can also be paired with magnesium threonate to promote healthy sleep patterns.

- **Chamomile tea:** Grandma knew what she was doing when she made chamomile tea before bed. Chamomile contains an antioxidant that binds to certain receptors in your brain to promote sleepiness.

- **Cannabis and/or CBD:** While still controversial (and illegal in some states), more and more perimenopausal and menopausal women are turning to cannabis to relieve their symptoms, according to a 2020 North American Menopause Society study.[102] Since there are no conclusive studies, experts recommend asking your health care provider if cannabis might be a viable option to help with your symptoms.[103] Many women also turn to CBD to help with sleep. CBD is similar to cannabis but without the THC, the chemical that gets you high. While there is no clear-cut evidence that CBD can relieve all menopausal symptoms, according to *Medical News Today*, there are some promising studies that show higher doses of CBD may help with sleep.[104]

- **Mushrooms,** yes, mushrooms! Medicinal mushrooms such as lion's mane or reishi can help both calm the mind and increase the duration of sleep.[105] There are some great mushroom teas and supplements out there that can really improve sleep. Just make sure they are from a reputable source.

Always consult with your doctor before you try any dietary supplement.

Exercise. Exercise. Exercise.

Yes! Exercise is an important part of self-care. We all know exercise is important for overall health, and regular exercise will also help promote restful sleep in the evening. Statistics show that 80% of Americans don't get enough exercise for optimal health.[106] Many people don't exercise because they don't think they have enough time, but did you know the recommended minimal amount of exercise is only twenty minutes per day? When you look at it that way, it's pretty doable!

BENEFITS OF REGULAR EXERCISE

- Lowers risk of heart disease and high blood pressure
- Helps regulate weight by supporting a healthy metabolism
- Slows the aging process by increasing bone density and helping to maintain muscle integrity
- Lowers risk of type 2 diabetes
- Lowers cholesterol
- Helps protect the body from various cancers
- Improves cognition and sleep
- Dopamine from exercise helps reduce anxiety and depression
- Lowers the risk of dementia and helps with brain health and memory
- You will have more energy!

There is so much research on how critical exercise is to healthy aging. The menopausal years come with physical changes like decreased bone density, decreased muscle mass, and an increased risk of chronic health issues such as heart disease and osteoporosis. Exercise is not only a crucial component to maintaining physical health; there are mental benefits as well. So many of our clients and friends have told us if they didn't exercise, they would go nuts!

We are sure you have seen the pharmaceutical ads for osteoporosis. But here are the facts: Menopausal women have an increased risk for osteoporosis due to dropping estrogen levels. Exercise, especially weight-bearing exercise, is so important for women in midlife.

You don't have to spend hours at the gym or hire an expensive trainer to move your body, and it doesn't have to be time-consuming either. Try simple things like taking the stairs and parking in the furthest spot from the door to get extra steps in. It can be ten minutes here and ten minutes there. Just move! Here are some of the best exercises for midlife women:

- **Weight-bearing exercises:** Body-weight exercises like walking, jogging, and dancing are great because they help maintain and even increase bone density, which reduces the risk for osteoporosis. You might even consider investing in a weighted vest for walking to counteract the effects of hormonal changes in muscle mass and bone density.

- **Strength training:** You can use weights, resistance bands, or even body weight to build and maintain muscle mass, which decreases with age and hormonal changes. After age fifty, we drop 1-2% of muscle mass each year, and that increases to 3% over age sixty.[107] Weight training not only prevents muscle deterioration but helps to rebuild it.

- **Low-impact exercises** like swimming, cycling, and yoga: These exercises can help improve cardiovascular health and flexibility and don't put excessive strain on joints.

- **Pelvic-floor exercises:** Here's one not many women are told about. Pelvic-floor exercises and doing Kegels properly (see our sex chapter) are so important, especially in midlife, because the pelvic-floor muscles tend to weaken during this time. Do these to help with urinary incontinence.

- **Stress-reducing exercises:** You can put yoga in this category too, but what we're talking about here are things like deep breathing, meditation, and tai chi. These are great for relaxation!

Other exercises you might consider are tennis, pickleball, barre, Pilates, hula hooping (it's super fun!), hiking, spinning, boxing, cross training, Tabata, bike-riding, rollerblading, skiing, stand-up paddleboarding, snowshoeing, jumping rope, kayaking . . . the list goes on and on.

Pam

I'll be honest here and tell you I hated PE in high school. I didn't like running, and I was a pretty uncoordinated athlete. My high school gym teachers would be shocked at what I do now! I love weight lifting and spin cycling and regularly take classes like Shred or Barbell. Crazy, right? On the other hand, who can do hardcore all the time? So I balance my exercise by also doing Pilates and yoga, and on nice weekends, I love getting out for a bike ride. Exercise has become a non-negotiable part of my life because I feel so much better when I do it.

That lucky bitch Julie got out of PE in high school by taking an extra academic class instead. Kinda nerdy, but she got out of wearing the Catholic school gym uniforms that were not chic! She has always loved yoga and is passionate about swimming. Julie relishes the warm months when she can swim outside. In Chicago, that's April to November (brrrr. . . maybe a bit chilly then!). She sometimes swims when it's snowing, but she loves it, and it feeds her soul. Bonus: Cold water helps with inflammation, boosts the immune system, and burns a lot of calories. Super bonus: Cold water improves libido.[108] Julie has waterproof earbuds and also uses her swimming time to listen to meditative music. Talk about two-for-one multitasking!

Us

Don't be frustrated if you don't see the benefits of exercise right away. On average, it takes around twelve weeks to notice a difference in your physical body.[109] Just stay focused on the other benefits of exercise, like how you are sleeping, how you feel mentally, and how it lowers your stress levels and improves your posture.

Make regular exercise a priority—because you're worth it, and your body will thank you in the long run. The important thing is to find the type of movement and exercise that speak to you so that you will do it. Look at exercise like a buffet; there are so many choices, and doing anything is better than doing nothing. If you're new, start small. Take a ten-minute walk, find a ten-minute yoga routine on YouTube, or lift small hand weights. Your body will thank you!

As with any exercise program, it's important to consult with a health care professional before starting it to ensure the exercises are safe and appropriate for you!

Self-care extends beyond the physical realm. You can eat healthy, drink water, and exercise, but keep in mind that self-care encompasses caring for your emotional and mental states as well. These next few suggestions address that.

Practice Gratitude

This is an often overlooked form of self-care. Gratitude has the power to not only enrich your life, but can also completely elevate your well-being. If you allow it, gratitude can become a way of life, a mindset that can bring immense joy and contentment.

We already discussed living in a fast-paced modern world, and part of that world is the consumer-driven society—it's so easy to get caught up in the pursuit of more. More everything: possessions, achievements, recognition. It's seriously exhausting, and you may have all the stuff but still feel the desire for the next thing. Gratitude allows you time to stop the cycle and invites you to just pause, take a breath, reflect on the present moment, and appreciate all that already surrounds you.

When you take the time to embrace a grateful mindset, you open your eyes to the beauty of life, even amid difficulties. You might see silver linings, the blessing of the lessons, and opportunities for growth and expansion.

We want to share a story about the power of gratitude. We had a client, Amy, who came to us because she was constantly tired and couldn't lose weight despite eating healthy and having a solid exercise routine. After several sessions, we noticed she tended to focus on what was lacking in her life and compared herself to others. It became clear that Amy was feeling deeply unfulfilled in her life and that the weight she was carrying wasn't due to diet or exercise. We had her limit her time on social media and start a gratitude journal to write three things down each morning and each evening that she was grateful for—even if it was the smallest thing. She was resistant at first but trusted in the process and initially began writing down little things like coffee, the sun, and her bed. After a while, something magical happened. We could see her energy shift. Her eyes were brighter, there was a spring in her step, and she was even sleeping better. Amy noticed the kindness of strangers, the beauty of nature, and even the health she enjoyed, which she had taken for granted. Not only did her relationships improve, but she started sleeping better and had a ton more energy. It was powerful to bear witness to such a powerful transformation from such a seemingly small shift.

There is a lot of great research on gratitude that shows benefits for your mental, emotional, and even physical wellness. Gratitude is linked to increased happiness, reduced stress, improved relationships, enhanced self-esteem, and better overall mental health.[110] [111] A regular gratitude practice can rewire your brain! It shifts your focus from negativity to positivity and appreciation.

Like with exercise, you can start small. You can keep a little journal by the bed as our client did and just write down three things you are grateful for (morning and night if you can). It's wonderful to start your day with a grateful mindset and to wind down your day by reflecting on the good things that happened to you. It can be as simple as being grateful you have a cozy bed and a nice home or that you have a prized parking spot.

The best thing about gratitude is that it's free, and you can do it at any time. It's an invitation to slow down and see what is around you. It can be as simple as appreciating your senses, the beauty of a sunrise or sunset, laughter shared with friends, the food on your plate, or clean drinking water. We invite you to take a few moments before bed and write down three things you were grateful for that day. We promise your life will change.

Spend Time in Nature

Let's face facts here. Most of us are living in a fast-paced, technology centered world. Taking some time to be in nature can be one of the most powerful, yet perhaps most overlooked, forms of self-care.

If you allow it, nature can give you a full-body reset. When you step outside, your senses come alive. Just feel the sun on your skin, listen to the sound of birds, enjoy the scents of trees or flowers. What happens? It's as if all of a sudden, you are out of your head and into the present moment. This natural (and free!) form of mindfulness calms the nervous system, lowers cortisol levels, and helps ease anxiety and stress.

According to Harvard health, just spending 20 minutes in nature can help lower hormone stress levels.[112] The American Heart Association says it can improve mood, enhance focus, and reduce blood pressure.[113] Whether it's a walk in the woods, a few moments of deep breathing under a tree, your feet in the sand, or some time just relaxing on your patio, nature acts as a quiet yet powerful healer.

Have you ever heard of grounding or earthing? Think of walking outside barefoot in the sand or grass, or lying on the ground in the backyard —it's when your body has physical contact with the earth. Our earth has an electric charge and when your body comes into direct contact with it, it naturally absorbs that charge which may have a number of health benefits.

Historically, humans were more connected to earth. We spent a lot of time outside and slept on natural surfaces. But today we just don't have that same contact because of shoes and spending so much time in indoor spaces. Plus these days we are constantly connected to some form of technology. What happens is our bodies build up a positive static electric charge that can't be released unless we connect to the ground. Grounding has been shown to improve sleep, heal wounds and reduce inflammation.[114]

Walking or touching the ground isn't the only way you can ground yourself. Today, there are special shoes that can keep you grounded, sheets and mats that plug into an outlet and products that plug directly into the ground. You know that little round hole above the two little rectangles on your outlets? That is the ground on your outlet and it connects directly to the earth! Interesting, right?

As midlife women, time spent in nature or grounding can be a powerful reconnection point—physically, spiritually, and emotionally. It creates space to reflect, release, and re-center. Plus, it's free, accessible, and deeply restorative.

Personal Growth and Development

This may also be an often-overlooked form of self-care. Everyone, not just midlife women, has the innate need for growth and personal development. It's how we learn to become the best versions of ourselves, and it is a key factor in having a fulfilling life.

When you pursue growth, you open up endless possibilities to expand your horizons, broaden your perspectives, and gain new knowledge and skills. And when you choose new activities that may be outside your comfort zone, you stimulate your mind and promote intellectual growth, which is so important as we age!

We are both lifelong learners. We love taking new classes, whether they be about cooking, exercising, or even how to write a book! We both have stacks of books by the bed. But if you were one of those kids who hated school, it doesn't have to be so structured now that you are a grown-up. You could take some higher education classes, learn a new hobby, take up a new instrument, or learn about a new technology. Even reading this book is personal growth, as is anything that keeps you curious about the world around you.

We are going to encourage you to check out your community or local college—the classes they offer now are fascinating, and many of them are at a nominal cost. It makes us want to be in college again! There are also a lot of online courses, both free and paid. Masterclass, Coursera, Futurelearn, and Kadenza are a great place to start, and even schools like Harvard offer online classes.

You might ask why this is important for self-care. While growth and personal development are great for contributing to your emotional well-being and resilience, they are also great for enhancing self-esteem and for even meeting new people, which we know is hard to do as we get older.

Having a Purpose

Wait. Having a purpose is self-care? Yes! We have found that many midlife women feel like they are wandering around, feeling a bit lost. Especially if they have been caring for children or parents and now have free time or are making career transitions or shifts in relationships. Midlife marks a period of profound personal growth and self-reflection. Having some direction and purpose is like having a compass to guide you. Many women experience a natural inclination to reassess their lives and seek deeper meaning. It's a great opportunity to discover new interests, passions, and desires that align with your authentic self.

Midlife women have the advantage of wisdom and life experience. Think of all the challenges you've overcome, the lessons you've learned, and the many skills you've acquired. This is the time to reflect on all those things and draw upon your experiences to shape a meaningful future. Your life isn't over at midlife!

Some women struggle with this, and it can come with challenges. It might mean embracing change, stepping outside your comfort zone, and challenging societal expectations. You might need to overcome fears and self-doubt, but the journey is different for everyone. When you have a purpose, you are driven by a sense of calling, a higher mission that goes beyond just gain. It is not uncommon for midlife women to completely change careers to pursue something they feel called to or passionate about.

Finding your purpose is a deeply introspective activity. If you don't know where to start, here are some ideas that might help you find something you resonate with:

SELF-REFLECTION

- Journaling your thoughts, dreams, and aspirations can help you uncover things that bring you joy and fulfillment.

- Meditating, which is also great for stress, helps you quiet your mind and focus inward and can give clarity to your true desires and passions

- Ask yourself open-ended questions like, "What are my core values?" "What brings me joy?" "What impact do I want to have in the world?" Sit quietly and see what comes up for you.

EXPLORE YOUR PASSIONS AND INTERESTS

- Step out of your comfort zone and try a new hobby, sport, or even volunteering!

- Take a class or workshop on something you have always been interested in.

SEEK OUT INSPIRATION

- Try reading biographies of women that inspire you.

- There are so many great podcasts created by midlife women who are only just finding purpose. One of them may inspire you.

SEEK SUPPORT

- If you are thinking about a career shift, seek out a career counselor.

- Join women's groups to connect with other women also on the journey. *Midlife Upgrade* has a community, and Meetup is another place to go.

Connection

Finding support and connection becomes vital in midlife. There is a study done by the *Industrial Psychiatry Journal* published in *Psychology Today* that shows a significant relationship between depression and loneliness in older people (not that we are old).[115] We do know female friendships are important and are the key to happiness for women. And we also know midlife women, in particular, are seeking community and connection because they have told us. Because this is such an important topic, we are going to go into it much deeper in the chapter on relationships.

One of the most important connections you can have is with yourself. We started this chapter by saying self-care *is* self-love. Here's a quick exercise to bring you back to a place of self-love in an instant no matter how stressed you feel:

- Simply close your eyes, put your hand on your heart, and breathe into that area.

- Then silently ask yourself the question, "What's the most loving thing I could do for myself right now?"

Self-Care Mastery

You can be doing all the "right stuff" but still lack the energy and vitality you are seeking. Sometimes it's not only about what you add in, but also about what you take out. Toxicity can come in unexpected ways. When you remove these "toxins" from your life, you open space for more light and love:

- **Toxic people:** There are people who suck the energy right out of you—energy vampires. You are the combination of the five people you spend the most time with. Choose to only surround yourself with people that lift you and light you up.

- **Complaining:** Fun fact—complaining releases cortisol.[116] It physically stresses you out. If that's not enough to get you to stop, it also attracts more negativity. The next time you feel a complaint coming on, take a breath and turn that complaint into a positive statement. We will give you an example: Let's say your car breaks down. Instead of saying, "I can't believe my car is broken," say instead, "I am so lucky to have a car."

- **Gossiping:** When you gossip, you not only hurt others, you hurt yourself. Toxic gossiping has the same effect as complaining and it brings your integrity into question.

- **Criticizing:** Criticizing others is not going to lead them to change their behavior, and in the end, it just feeds a lose-lose situation. Instead of criticizing, offer your love, support, or guidance.

- **Being Negative:** Believe it or not, negativity can lead to a weakened immune system.[117] The body doesn't lie. And constant negativity can easily spiral into doom and gloom. While not everything is rainbows and unicorns, notice when you are having an ANT (automatic negative thought) and replace it with a positive affirmation. This requires some self-awareness and practice, but over time, you will begin to attract more goodness.

- **Making Excuses:** This is a good one. It's easy to shrug off responsibility. While we can't always control what happens to us, we *always* have the ability to choose how we respond. We often make excuses out of fear or uncertainty, but once you take personal responsibility, you will find that only you control your future.

- **Toxic Thoughts:** We cannot stress enough how important it is to be mindful (pun intended) of your thoughts. Start noticing when you have negative thoughts, especially about yourself! Did you know 60-80% of your thoughts are negative?[118] If you are constantly having negative thoughts about yourself, imagine what this is doing to your mental and physical health. In his book, *Change Your Brain, Change Your Body*, Dr. Daniel Amen discusses in detail ANTS (automatic negative thoughts) and how to minimize them to improve your health. Just being aware you have them can help with making a change. Speak to yourself as you would a good friend.

We have by no means covered everything there is to cover on self-care and could write a whole book on this topic alone. But we recognize that in the busy world we live in, self-care is often the first thing women neglect. We hope that we have given you some ideas to bring your awareness back to yourself and some areas in your life that might need attention. Remember that this journey is a marathon, not a sprint. Be patient with yourself and celebrate the small wins toward prioritizing your well-being. Once you start to shift your perspective toward knowing self-care is an essential act of self-love, not only will you thrive, but you will ultimately uplift those around you. We promise!

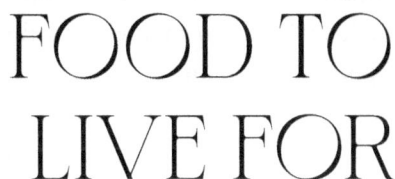

CHAPTER 6

FOOD TO LIVE FOR

"Eat food. Not too much. Mostly plants."
—Michael Pollan

This quote by Michael Pollan is one of our favorites. Both of us have tried it all: paleo, raw, macrobiotic, vegetarian, vegan, and more. Pam is also certified as a raw-food and vegan chef. And both of our bookshelves are filled with an abundance of cookbooks because we *love* food. We have learned from experimenting with ourselves and working with clients that no one diet is perfect for everyone, and some extreme diets (like raw) have diminishing returns. We also learned that we can have the most optimal diet in the world and still not feel well—because it's not always about the food.

Pam

In my twenties, I used to pretty much be able to eat and drink whatever I wanted and maintain my health and weight. I became interested in health and nutrition at around thirty when I became pregnant with my daughter. I knew I was only going to have one child, so I set out to learn all that I could about healthy nutrition and lifestyle. The book that started me on my life-long journey to learn about health was *Diet for a New America* by John Robbins. After devouring (pun intended) that book, I began choosing healthy foods, taking cooking classes and courses, exercising more regularly, and studying various dietary theories. I also became a certified holistic health coach. All of these things completely took my health to another level. But once I turned fifty, all bets were off! I put on weight out of the blue, and eating mostly vegan wasn't doing it for me. At this stage of life, I had to rethink what was optimal for me and started incorporating more protein into my diet. But—and I want to stress this—it's not one-size-fits-all.

Today, I eat more of a Mediterranean diet, and I feel much more balanced. Extreme diet plans don't seem to work well for me. While I still eat heavily plant-based, I now incorporate more lean, clean fish and animal protein into my diet.

Julie

In my twenties (a lifetime ago), I had a boyfriend who owned a super popular health food store in New York City. Decades before Whole Foods, it was a mecca for all things health and wellness in Manhattan. And like Pam, I, too, read *Diet for a New America* and was blown away by the information. I became a vegetarian, and my favorite restaurants were macrobiotic. I was super healthy. But after a scuba diving trip to Mexico, I started having serious gastrointestinal issues. I was losing weight rapidly. My mother came across an article—*the universe is always working in our favor!*—about a brilliant Brazilian parasitologist MD, practicing in NYC, who had patented a simple test capable of detecting many different types of parasites. He was able to diagnose and treat me with herbs from the Amazon. (FYI, he told me never to eat sushi, so that's usually off my menu!) When I moved to Chicago, home of the stockyards and a meat-eating city, I began eating a more varied diet and incorporated some animal protein. Now, in midlife, I am doing my best to eat adequate amounts of protein with plenty of vegetables. I usually eat pretty simply: I enjoy a morning green smoothie and have some type of protein with every meal, although I just don't crave red meat much anymore. I also usually "fast" for fourteen hours between dinner and breakfast. I love eating delicious food—my son is an amazing cook and a total foodie, so new restaurants are often on the agenda. And then all bets are off. I'll try anything.

Us

In this chapter, we are going to talk about foods that feed your body and what feeds your soul so that you can feel amazing from the inside out and shine like the star you are.

Our food sources in the twenty-first century aren't what they were for our grandparents. Pam's grandparents grew a lot of their food, had chickens, baked bread, and canned for the winter. Today, to have optimal health, we have to be more mindful about where our food comes from and the life force it has. Food today is grown with toxic pesticides; it is picked before it's ripe, sprayed with chemicals to make it ripen, and doesn't have peak nutritional value. Many foods are now hybridized or genetically modified. We have become a culture of convenience, and people often eat prepackaged or pre-made foods, which can also be laden with chemicals.

Okay, so what does this have to do with menopause? Well, during the midlife years, some women find themselves gaining weight even though they may not be eating any more than usual (or maybe even eating less). Some women weigh the same as they have for years, but their shape begins to change—they have more fat around the belly, fuller breasts, curvier hips, and less muscle tone. Some women also say they feel hungry. All. The. Time. What the heck is going on?! Here are some of the reasons for midlife weight gain:

INSULIN RESISTANCE

Insulin is an essential hormone (yes, another hormone!) produced by the pancreas that helps to turn food into energy and regulate blood sugar levels. A diet high in refined carbs like sugar, white flour, and alcohol can cause your cells to become insulin-resistant. Your pancreas has to pump out more and more insulin into your cells as a response to sugar overload.

Over time, your cells stop responding, and the pancreas just can't keep up.[119] So your blood sugar keeps rising, which means those delicious carbs are just converting to fat. Quickly. Around the middle. This tends to catch up with us in midlife.

XENOESTROGENS

Have you ever heard of this word? If not, you need to know it. Xenoestrogens are molecules that closely resemble estrogen and are found in things like plastics, cleaning products, pesticides, perfumes, cosmetics, store receipts, and ... the list goes on and on. They come from man-made industrial compounds like BPA, PCB, and phthalates, and they stimulate the cells with estrogen receptors—for example, breast tissue and uterine endometrial tissue. There is a full list in our book portal. The really bad thing about xenoestrogens is your body doesn't know the difference between the endogenous (real) estrogen it makes and the fake toxic estrogen. Xenoestrogens are huge hormone disruptors that can completely throw your hormones out of balance and cause toxic weight gain, especially around the middle.[120]

Many women suffer from this and have absolutely no idea. And we are especially sensitive and vulnerable to these chemicals. Your estrogen levels can test normal or even low; however, you may have estrogen dominance due to an excess of xenoestrogens in your body. Xenoestrogens are not detectable by measuring estrogen levels in the blood, saliva, or urine, yet they act like estrogen in the body. The only way to find out if you have any xenoestrogens in your body is to test for each toxin by using environmental toxin testing. Many integrative and functional medicine practitioners provide this type of testing. This is a key thing for midlife women to know.

MENOPAUSE

As estrogen levels wildly fluctuate during perimenopause and then drop off in menopause, proteins that cause fat cells to store even more fat are activated. These cellular changes slow down the fat-burning process, causing your body to shift fat storage to ... you guessed it ... your middle.[121] Dang it—we can't win.

ADRENAL HORMONAL IMBALANCE

We live in stressful times. Once upon a time, our stresses were few and far between, and our adrenals served us well. If you had to run from a bear, your adrenals kicked in, gave your body a burst of cortisol (energy), and allowed you to outrun the bear, store fat, and conserve your energy. As we discussed earlier, cortisol is the stress hormone that is produced by your adrenal glands, two little glands that sit atop your kidneys.[122] But beyond just cortisol, these glands produce multiple hormones and chemicals, which can also fall out of balance if your adrenals are stressed. They are responsible for regulating your stress response by controlling metabolism, inflammation, heart rate, blood pressure, blood sugar, and sleep patterns.[123]

In today's world, many of us are in constant fight-or-flight stress, and our adrenals are stressed! Stressed out adrenals cause low energy, a craving for sugar, salt and/or refined carbs to get more energy, and you guessed it . . . unfortunately, fat around the middle.

ENVIRONMENTAL TOXINS

We live in a world where we are bombarded with environmental toxins daily. Women especially! Since World War II, over 85,000 man-made chemicals have been registered just in the United States alone, and fewer than 1% have been tested for safety by the Environmental Protection Agency.[124] We are bombarded by chemicals before we even leave the house—water from the shower, lotions, hair-care products, makeup, perfumes, and pesticides in and on our food.

According to Dr. Mark Hyman, one of our favorite functional-medicine doctors, these chemicals cause inflammation, create hormonal imbalances, and overload our natural detoxification systems.[125] What does this all have to do with weight gain? While the liver is responsible for cleansing these toxins from our body, sooner or later, it becomes sluggish and impaired due to overloading. He says that when toxins can no longer be eliminated, they are stored in body fat to be dealt with at a later date, usually in the form of some mystery illness. The fat is protecting your vital organs by trapping these harmful toxins. So the more toxins we ingest, the greater need for more fat and . . . weight gain. If you don't pay attention to what you're putting on or in your body, you will have a more difficult time maintaining a healthy weight, especially in midlife. That's why we are also going to include information on detoxification in this chapter.

Women in midlife who aren't managing their diet and lifestyle are at a much higher risk for metabolic diseases such as obesity, diabetes, high blood pressure, heart disease, and other issues such as breast, uterine, and endometrial cancers, polycystic ovary syndrome, overstimulation of ovarian testosterone (excess hair on face; hair loss on scalp), and adult acne. Years of eating too many refined carbs, lack of exercise, and exposure to toxins may finally catch up to us in midlife.

Nutrition 101

First of all, let's talk about carbohydrates, which are one of the macronutrients your body requires. Not all carbohydrates are bad! In fact, they are your body's main source of energy. However, not all carbs are equal or do the same thing in the body. We like to tell our clients that 100 calories of broccoli in the body is very different from 100 calories of potato chips. It's not about the calories; it's about the quality of the calories. Many women turn to simple carbs for energy. Chocolate cake, anyone?

Simple carbohydrates like sugar, white flour, and high-fructose corn syrup can not only raise your blood sugar levels but also zap your energy. If you eat a bagel for breakfast, we guess that you are going to crave some coffee mid-morning because your blood sugar will crash. It's a vicious cycle. These foods are also generally devoid of any fiber that would help to slow down the release of sugars that are absorbed into your bloodstream. The other thing about simple carbs is they tend to be calorie-dense. While we are not so much about counting calories, it's the type of calories you eat that matters!

Complex carbohydrates are what your body wants and needs! Think fresh fruits and vegetables, sea vegetables, unrefined grains, and legumes. Eating foods like these will give you energy and keep your blood sugar levels in check.

Fats, like carbohydrates, are not all bad, and they are also a macronutrient your body needs. Back in the 1960s, the American Heart Association told us fats were "bad" for heart health, and many fake fats, like shortening and margarine, flooded the market.[126] These types of fats are detrimental to your health! But the truth is, you do need *healthy* fat in your diet. Fat gives us energy and is stored for later use when the energy we use from carbohydrates is exhausted. Fat is also the basic component of cell membranes in every cell in your body! It is a crucial nutrient for body growth and development. And fat helps us absorb vitamins like A, D, E, and K. The type of fat you consume affects your weight and impacts your overall health.

Trans fats are hands-down one of the worst things you can put in your body. Seriously. These are the fats that raise the bad cholesterol and lower the good cholesterol. These are man-made fats created when hydrogen is added to vegetable oils to make them solid at room temperature so they last longer and don't spoil as quickly. Gross, right? These fats can increase your likelihood of heart disease, and fortunately, some countries are banning them. However, you can still find trans fats in microwave popcorn, shortening, margarine, fried foods, frozen pizza, and non-dairy creamer—just to name a few. Even though the FDA in the United States has banned trans fats, they can still be sneaked into many processed foods. If the food contains a half-gram of trans fat or less per serving, you won't even see it listed on the label. We recommend avoiding any overly processed foods.

Saturated fats are the fats mostly found in animal foods like dairy products—butter, ice cream, milk, and cheese—fatty cuts of beef or pork, eggs, cured meats, and even chicken skin. However, they are also in some plant-based foods like coconut oil and palm kernel oil. These are fats that should be consumed sparingly. There is a lot of conflicting information out there around saturated fats, and even within this category, the type of saturated fat makes a difference. If you are going to consume saturated fat, quality matters, so read your labels. Look for foods that say grass-fed, pasture-raised, or organic coconut oil if you choose to consume these foods.

Unsaturated fats are fats that are liquid at room temperature. And they are the good fats! These are the fats that can lower bad cholesterol and raise good cholesterol. Even within this category, there are two types of unsaturated fats:

1. **Monounsaturated fats** are in some oils such as olive and peanut oils, as well as avocados, nuts like almonds and pecans, and some seeds, like pumpkin and sesame seeds.

2. **Polyunsaturated fats** are found in some oils, including soybean and grapeseed oils. They are also in flaxseed, walnuts, and fish like salmon. Most of us don't eat enough of these good fats, so we included some recipes in our book portal so that you can incorporate more of these good fats into your diet.

Protein is the third and final macronutrient. Protein is an essential macronutrient because it helps to build and repair muscles and cells and fuel your body. It also helps with hormone regulation, so you need to make sure you are getting what your body needs, which varies from woman to woman.

At one time, we were both vegans. However, as we got older, we started to experience some fatigue and started having more cravings for animal foods. We listened to our bodies and started incorporating more grass-fed meats, pasture-raised chicken, and wild-caught, sustainable seafood into our diets and felt much better! But you should know there are also proteins in vegetables. According to *EatingWell* magazine, the plant foods highest in protein are green peas, spinach, artichokes, sweet corn (get it organic!), avocado, asparagus, brussel sprouts, mushrooms, kale, and potatoes. Listen to your body because it knows! Your dietary needs will change as you age, and you may need to make modifications.

Here's the thing, though: Protein intake for midlife women is super important. As women age, we are at an increased risk for muscle loss due to hormonal changes. Protein protects muscle mass and muscle function and helps prevent osteopenia and osteoporosis. It's worth noting that the RDA (recommended daily allowance) for protein is 0.8 grams of protein per kilogram of body weight. That may not be enough! Dr. Mary Clair

Haver, author of *The New Menopause*, recommends 1.5 to 1.8 grams per kilogram of body weight, and she even has a handy protein calculator that you can find in our resources.[127]

Now you may be wondering what the best balance of macronutrients is for optimal health. *Remember, the macronutrients are carbohydrates, fats, and proteins.* Generally speaking, aim for thirty to 35% healthy carbohydrates like fruits and veggies, 25-30% healthy fats like avocados, nuts, or seafood, and 35-40% lean protein like grass-fed meats, pastured chicken, organic tofu, yogurt, or quinoa.

There are some great apps for tracking your food. If you are struggling with your weight or lack of energy, we strongly encourage you to track your food intake. We do this with all new coaching clients. We find it helps them balance their macronutrients and raises their awareness of the quantity and quality of their food choices.

We 100% agree with the quote at the beginning of this chapter, "Eat food. Not too much. Mostly plants." If you're not familiar with Michael Pollan, he's an award-winning writer and journalist, and Pam first learned of him when she read his book *In Defense of Food: An Eater's Manifesto*. In the book, Pollan examines how much of the food we find in modern supermarkets, fast food chains, and restaurants isn't what his grandmother would recognize as real food. He discourages eating "edible food-like substances."

Some of you lucky women may have gotten away with eating pretty much whatever you like with little or no weight gain or issues with your health. This may catch up to you in midlife. While hormones play a part in midlife weight changes, years of eating refined carbs and drinking that evening glass of wine might finally have taken their toll.

MICHAEL POLLAN'S SEVEN RULES FOR EATING:[128]

1. Don't eat anything your great-grandmother wouldn't recognize as food. "When you pick up that box of portable yogurt tubes or eat something with 15 ingredients you can't pronounce, ask yourself, 'What are those things doing there?'"

2. Don't eat anything with more than five ingredients or ingredients you can't pronounce.

3. Stay out of the middle of the supermarket; shop on the perimeter. Real food (fruits and veggies) tends to be on the outer edge near the loading docks, where it can easily be replaced.

4. Don't eat anything with an expiration date in the next millennium. "There are exceptions, like honey —but as a rule, things like Twinkies that never go bad aren't food," Oh, the days when we ate Twinkies!

5. It is not just what you eat but how you eat. "Always leave the table a little hungry," Pollan says. "Many cultures have rules that you stop eating before you are full. In Japan, they say eat until you are four-fifths full. Islamic culture has a similar rule, and in German culture, they say, 'Tie off the sack before it's full.'"

6. Families traditionally ate together, around a table and not a TV, at regular meal times. It's a good tradition. It's very nourishing to eat meals with the people you love.

7. Don't buy food where you buy your gasoline. Most of what is in convenience stores is inedible, meaning it is *not* healthy for you. And in the United States, 20% of food is eaten in the car.

While all of these rules are beneficial, we would also like to address eating on the go and eating alone. Which a lot of us do now. Research shows eating in a community can be healthier than eating alone—both physically and psychologically. A 2015 study in the journal *Appetite* found that people who eat alone tend to have poorer eating habits than those who sit down at a table and eat with others.[129] When we eat in a community, we tend to eat more fruits and vegetables. Eating with others is good for stress levels because it helps us to relax and creates positive feelings of love and connection, activating the parasympathetic nervous system and helping with digestive function.

So, the big bonus is that eating with our family and friends—in community—promotes healthier aging. Telomeres are DNA structures found at both ends of each chromosome, and they are markers that indicate your rate of aging. One of the ways to keep your telomeres healthy is by eating a diet full of unprocessed, whole foods like fruits, vegetables, and legumes, and as we said, we tend to eat healthier when we eat with others.

So you may be thinking, "Let's get to it!" What is the best diet? Research shows that eating a Mediterranean diet is one of the healthiest diets on the planet.[130] It's great for weight loss, longevity, heart health, and disease prevention, but best of all, it's one of the easiest diets to follow long-term as part of a healthy lifestyle! The Mediterranean diet includes foods like fruits and vegetables, legumes, whole grains, fresh herbs and spices, and olive oil. Seafood rich in omega-3 fatty acids is also encouraged—think salmon, sardines, and tuna. Just make sure your seafood is from a clean source (you may have to speak with your fishmonger about this). Foods high in saturated fats, like chicken, turkey, red meat, butter, yogurt, and eggs are used sparingly.

You may have also heard of the Blue Zones. The blue zones are five regions in the world that author Dan Buettner identified as areas where people not only live the longest but are also the healthiest.[131] Interestingly enough, two of these regions are located in the Mediterranean: Sardinia, Italy, and Ikara, Greece. People in these regions eat pretty similarly to how Michael Pollan believes we should eat. We highly recommend you check Buettner's cookbook, *The Blue Zones Kitchen*, as it has some wonderful, healthy recipes.

Breakfast (or break the fast) can be as simple as smashed avocado and sprouts with a drizzle of olive oil on sourdough bread and some fresh fruit. Lunch can be a simple leafy green salad with fresh veggies and hummus. And dinner can be just a piece of grilled fish with roasted vegetables.

Here's the thing: It's not just about calories in, calories out. As we said earlier, your body responds very differently to 100 calories of potato chips than it does to 100 calories of broccoli. Since the Mediterranean diet emphasizes nutrient-dense foods, you may naturally find yourself eating (and craving) less over time. You are feeding your body the food it truly desires. Interestingly, some foods on the Mediterranean diet are calorically dense, like olive oil and nuts, so it's important to be mindful of how much of them you incorporate into your diet. While this diet is not a panacea for immediate weight loss, if you follow it over time, you should find yourself having overall optimal health.

Some people aren't able to digest or tolerate grains, which are allowed on the Mediterranean diet. Dr. Mark Hyman coined the term "pegan" to describe a diet that is a combination of paleo and vegan and does not include grains. The benefit of following Dr. Hyman's pegan approach is that it is high in fruits and vegetables and in good quality fats. It is low on the glycemic index because it excludes sugar, flour, and refined carbohydrates. He also promotes organic, non-GMO, and, if possible, locally-grown fresh produce, grass-fed free-range meat, and low-mercury fish. Some people do very well on Hyman's pegan diet![132]

Keep in mind that no diet is one-size-fits-all, and food is such a personal decision. Also, in our experience, dietary needs change as we age, so make choices that complement your unique health conditions and preferences.

Let's review two diet programs that are very popular right now, keto and Whole30:

KETOGENIC DIET

The keto, or ketogenic, diet is a low-carb, high-fat way of eating. The premise is that the body is deprived of glucose (sugar)—which is the main source of energy for cells—and that the body instead uses fat for energy. On this plan, seventy to 90% of calories comes from fat, 5-20% comes from protein, and only 5% comes from carbohydrates. The idea is to shift your metabolism to a fat-burning machine, which in turn will allow you to lose the stubborn weight you may have been holding on to for years. It also promises better brain function and decreased inflammation. Sounds great, right?

But does it work? It sure does, and research shows there are benefits to lowering carb intake.[133] However, the average keto dieter may be eating a lot of processed meats, bacon, cheese, and dairy from factory-farmed animals. Many of these foods are loaded with antibiotics and hormones. The keto diet also allows fake sweeteners like aspartame, sucralose, and diet sodas, which are linked to other health problems. As long as it's low carb, it's allowed. Many keto dieters focus on macronutrients over food quality. We also know that a diet high in animal fats is taxing on the liver, and people who have had a cholecystectomy (gallbladder removal) might suffer severe stomach issues because it is harder for the body to digest and process fats without a gallbladder.

Some of the benefits of keto include reduced appetite, weight loss, increased levels of "good" cholesterol (HDL), improved levels of "bad" cholesterol (LDL), a decrease in blood sugar and insulin levels, and lower blood pressure. It has also been shown to be very healing for some brain disorders (epilepsy, just to name one). Midlife women, in particular, have found it to be helpful for the weight loss aspect, especially abdominal fat, which tends to be hard to lose.

Keto does *not* have to be all meat and cheese. There are healthier ways to do it. One of the biggest benefits of keto is the elimination of sugar. Sugar can cause all sorts of problems, not just weight gain. There are plenty of recipes for vegetarian and even vegan keto dieters. The idea is to limit carb intake while increasing healthy fats such as fish, meat, eggs, avocados, clean oils, and nuts. This isn't a diet book, so we encourage you to do your research because of bio-individuality. It's just another option if you are looking to lose a few pounds in midlife.

WHOLE30

The other hot diet is Whole30. Pam has personally done this diet. Here are the basics: You can have meat, seafood, eggs, vegetables, and natural fats, but you avoid sugar, alcohol, grains, legumes, and dairy for thirty days. For our clients who are addicted to sugar and cheese (two of the most addictive foods), this diet *works*. If they follow the plan with no cheating, they will lose their cravings for sweets and dairy, drop a few pounds, and generally feel better.

Whole30 is great if you are doing it as recommended—for thirty days. But there can be drawbacks. First of all, it's just not sustainable if you want to live a normal life. The program emphasizes no cheats, and an all-or-nothing approach just isn't healthy long term, especially for people who have struggled with eating disorders. When deprived, some people will go off the deep end and overindulge once the program is over. Some people have reported stomach issues like constipation and food sensitivities after completing the program. And, like keto, overdoing it on processed, low-quality meats is just not good for long-term health and can contribute to type 2 diabetes, certain cancers, and heart disease, just to name a few.

Both keto and Whole30 don't allow beans. For keto dieters, beans are too high in carbohydrates. Whole30 dieters are told beans have something called "phytates" that can potentially block the absorption of calcium, iron, and magnesium. This isn't completely true, by the way. While beans do indeed contain phytates, when soaked before cooking and eaten as part of a balanced diet, this isn't an issue.[134] Interestingly enough, in the Blue Zones, the one common denominator for all of the centenarians is the consumption of some type of bean or legume. You do the math.

Something that has worked well for women looking to lose weight in midlife is intermittent fasting. Pam likes to call it intermittent feasting—it just sounds better! Basically, intermittent fasting (or feasting) is an eating pattern that cycles between periods of eating and periods of not eating. You may not realize it, but you are already doing this! When you sleep at night, you are fasting; this is why your morning meal is called breakfast. It's break fast. Fasting is not a new concept, and many religions have incorporated fasting as part of their rituals for literally centuries. Muslims during the month of Ramadan. Jews, Hindus, and Buddhists fast at various times during the year. Even within Christianity, there are fasting practices.

Intermittent fasting is great for several reasons. We talked a bit earlier about insulin sensitivity and how high insulin levels make it difficult to lose weight. Intermittent fasting can help improve insulin sensitivity and reduce insulin levels. The other thing that intermittent fasting does is improve autophagy. Think of autophagy as your cellular clean-up system.

It promotes a healthy immune system, helps slow down aging, and helps prevent disease. Intermittent fasting has also been shown to help with brain and heart health, inflammation, and weight control. Research shows that after fasting for twelve or more hours, you start using stored fat for energy versus glucose (sugar).[135]

There are several ways to do it. The most popular methods are:

- **16:8** (Fast for sixteen hours with an eight-hour eating window; you might skip breakfast.)

- **14:10** (Fast for fourteen hours with a ten-hour eating window.)

- **5:2** (Only consume 500 to 600 calories on two consecutive days or eat normally for five days, fast for two.)

- **Eat, stop, eat** (Fast for twenty-four hours once or twice a week.)

We have found that the 16:8 and 14:10 methods are the easiest and most doable for our midlife clients (and us) because we are mostly fasting overnight. We encourage you to find what works best for you and to work at it slowly. If you dive in head-first, not only will you not get the results you're looking for, but you might also end up super crabby! (We speak from experience.) If you have never tried intermittent fasting, the first thing you will want to do is choose your optimal eating window and work up to that. So, let's say you want to work up to an eight-hour eating window. Start with pushing your normal eating window by thirty minutes. If you normally have breakfast at 7:00 a.m., try 7:30 a.m. When you feel comfortable with that, add another thirty minutes and so on until you can fast for a full sixteen hours.

If you are on the 16:8 plan, if your first meal is at 9:00 a.m., your dinner would be at 5:00 p.m. Or, you could choose to skip breakfast, have your first meal at noon, and have dinner by 8:00 p.m. It's flexible, and you can decide what works best for you. If you choose to forgo breakfast, you can still enjoy water, coffee, or plain tea during your fasting time because hydration is super important while fasting. It's also important to note fasting *won't work* if you are choosing processed foods. Make sure you are eating healthy during your "feasting" times.

A personal note here: Pam has tried intermittent fasting cold turkey. She does not recommend this! "I was super irritable and probably intolerable to my family," she says. "So I went back to the drawing board and started pushing my eating window back by thirty minutes. I would do this for a week and then the next week and so on until I was at a full sixteen-hour fast. At first, I had decided I would have my first meal around 10:00 a.m. and have dinner around 6:00 p.m., which worked great; however, I like to work out in the morning and found myself dragging through my workouts. So, while I still do intermittent fasting, I now have breakfast at 8:00 a.m. and dinner at 5:00 p.m. Because the program is flexible, I can change it up when I don't work out and have dinner a bit later."

Cravings

When interviewing women for this book, comments about cravings kept coming up—and that they had intensified during this transition. Pam found that interesting because she could totally relate! She used to keep her salty popcorn and chocolate right next to each other. So if you have cravings, know you are not alone. And know that your cravings might be trying to tell you something.

We talk a lot about hormones in this book, but the truth is, if your hormones aren't in balance, your sleep and energy suffer, you will feel emotional, and . . . you will have cravings. Usually, in the form of sweet (for energy) or salty (for comfort). It's okay! You're allowed to have cravings; just be aware of what's going on so you don't go off the deep end and eat the bad things that will contribute to the menopausal middle.

If you are experiencing cravings before you eat that salted chocolate caramel, stop and ask yourself what's going on. Because with what we have learned, the cravings are not usually just about the food. Here's a good way to know if you are truly hungry or if you are just having an intense craving. If you are really hungry, ask yourself if an apple will satisfy you. If you are really hungry, an apple might sound pretty good. We use this little trick on ourselves as well, and the truth is many times, we aren't hungry at all, and it gives us a chance to step back before we make a poor decision. Take note that often when feeling hungry or having cravings, you might just need water. Drink a glass of water and see if your craving goes away!

Let's talk about those pesky hormone fluctuations. You already know that progesterone and estrogen decline during perimenopause and menopause, and this can have effects on two other important hormones—leptin, the satiety hormone, and ghrelin, the hunger hormone. Leptin signals the brain when the body has had enough food and promotes feelings of fullness. Ghrelin, on the other hand, is the hunger hormone because it stimulates appetite.

When your hormones are imbalanced, you may have a reduced sensitivity to leptin, and then your body doesn't know when you have consumed enough. You will have not only an increase in appetite but cravings for high-calorie or high-sugar foods. Ice cream, anyone? The other issue is the ghrelin hormone can increase, and you will frequently feel hungry. Imbalanced hormones also affect your taste perceptions, and you may find yourself drawn to foods you wouldn't normally eat. For example, some women may develop a strong preference for sweets because they may perceive sweet foods differently or need higher levels of sweets to feel satisfied. It's important to note here that the relationship between hormones, appetite regulation, and cravings is complex and can vary widely from person to person. Not all women will experience the same cravings or to the same extent, and other factors like lifestyle, stress levels, and personal choices also play a big role in cravings during midlife.

The main reason we have included information on cravings is so that you can begin to understand the impact hormonal changes have on appetite regulation and taste perceptions and make more informed dietary decisions during this transitional phase of life. By incorporating a more balanced and nutrient-dense diet, managing stress, and seeking outside support if needed, you can make the best choices for you to support your overall health and well-being.

Nutrigenomic Testing

Choosing what to eat can be daunting, so you may want to consider nutrigenomic testing. This type of testing is becoming more and more popular—and affordable! In a nutshell, nutrigenomic testing can show how foods and nutrients in your diet interact with your genes.

Practitioners are using nutrigenomic testing more and more to aid patients in individualized dietary choices. For example, this type of testing can tell you if you are more prone to craving sugar, how your body responds to caffeine, and even how certain foods may cause you to develop high blood pressure or diabetes.

While genetic testing is a tool for giving a more targeted approach to individual nutrition needs, it's not the only factor. Things like diet, exercise, sleep, and supplements can play a role as well. If this is something you are interested in, we recommend speaking to a practitioner familiar with this testing.

Microbiome

If you've been hearing about a healthy gut biome, there is a good reason. There is more and more evidence that shows having a healthy biome is the key to overall health.[16] Our gut is often referred to as our "second brain," and it plays a crucial role in overall health and well-being. Did you know your gut is composed of trillions of microorganisms? In fact, your microbiome has approximately ten pounds (yes, you read that right!) of microorganisms that perform a huge number of functions in your body. These include bacteria, viruses, and fungi that impact aspects of both physical and mental health. As research on the gut increases, scientists continue to uncover new roles of this microscopic community, revealing more understanding of its important influences on our health. There are several functions of the gut:

- **Aid in digestion and nutrient absorption:** A healthy gut promotes efficient digestion, reduces problems like bloating and constipation, and supports nutrient absorption.

- **Immune function:** A significant part of your immunity (two-thirds in fact) resides in your gut.[17] The gut also helps to modulate the immune system, which reduces the risk of infections, allergies, and autoimmune disorders.

- **Mental health:** There is a gut-brain axis, which is a bi-directional network between the gut and brain that influences mood, behavior, and cognitive function. Imbalance in the gut has been linked to depression, anxiety, and even Alzheimer's disease.

- **Metabolic health:** Certain bacteria in the gut help extract energy from our diet and regulate fat storage. A healthy gut is associated with better metabolic health, improved insulin sensitivity, and lowered risk of obesity-related diseases.

- **Inflammation and disease prevention:** Inflammation is a hot topic—and with good reason. Chronic inflammation is at the root of diseases like cardiovascular disease, diabetes, and even certain cancers. A healthy gut makes for lower inflammation.

Why talk about biome in a book about midlife and menopause? There is new research coming out that shows menopause can disrupt the microbiome.[136] A recent study in the journal *Menopause* showed a connection between energy and estrogen metabolism and menopause.[137] The study demonstrated that menopause may disrupt the microbiome, which can lead to fat gain, lower metabolism, and increased insulin resistance. So one way to improve metabolic health during the menopause transition may be through healing the gut.

If you notice you have begun to experience more bloating, constipation, stomach cramps, and gas, this may be why! What's a girl to do? Here are some suggestions:

Fiber: One of the best things you can do for gut health is eat more fiber. And the way you get more fiber is by eating more plant-based foods. If you can get your daily fiber intake up to thirty grams, your gut will thank you! Thirty grams is not that much, and to give you an idea, thirty grams looks like twelve pennies or a little less than a new pencil. Build your diet around fruits and vegetables, and you will have a happier tummy.

Fiber acts as a prebiotic, nourishing the beneficial bacteria in your gut and helping them thrive while preventing harmful bacteria from disrupting your microbiome. There are two types of fiber: soluble and insoluble. Soluble fiber dissolves in water and can be found in foods like oat bran, dried beans, peas, nuts, flaxseed, oranges, and apples. It promotes satiety, helping you feel fuller longer. Insoluble fiber, which doesn't dissolve in water, is found in whole grains like brown rice and wheat as well as in leafy greens, green beans, seeds, and nuts. It aids in waste elimination, detoxification, and maintaining bowel regularity.

Incorporating fiber-rich foods into your diet offers numerous benefits. Fiber enhances insulin sensitivity, regulates blood sugar levels, optimizes your gut microbiome, and reduces chronic inflammation. It also protects your intestines and colon, decreases the risk of depression, and supports overall digestive health. Making fiber a priority is an essential step toward a healthier, more balanced life.

Fermented foods: Fermented foods contain the good types of bacteria your gut loves. There's a reason fermented foods have been around for thousands of years. Try things like miso, sauerkraut, kimchi, pickled foods, low-sugar kombucha, and kefir. Yogurt can also be a good choice, but look for sugar-free varieties containing live bacteria.

Prebiotic foods: We hear a lot about probiotics, but good bacteria require prebiotics to thrive. Foods high in prebiotics are asparagus, apples, leeks, oatmeal, garlic, legumes, dandelion greens, barely ripe bananas, and Jerusalem artichokes.

Postbiotic foods: Oh yes, there is a third "biotic," and it's one you're going to be hearing more and more about. This is going to sound a bit strange, but postbiotics are basically the waste products from the probiotic bacteria, and yes, your gut needs them, too. Postbiotics produce butyrate in the lower gut and help boost the immune system, prevent leaky gut, and help with IBS. Foods that help with the production of butyrate are whole grains like brown rice or oats, legumes such as beans, lentils or chickpeas, vegetables, nuts, seeds, and even dark chocolate (just look for the high-quality, low-sugar variety).

Avoid artificial sweeteners: There are a lot of reasons to avoid artificial sweeteners, but when it comes to gut health, things like saccharin and aspartame are shown to disrupt the balance and diversity of gut bacteria.

Avoid anti-inflammatories: NSAIDS like aspirin or ibuprofen are known to upset the gut—it even says so on the package! Not only do they compromise the gut bacteria, but overuse can also erode the protective lining of the gut, leading to the condition known as "leaky gut."

Practice mindfulness: Here's one you may not have even considered. We talked earlier about fight-or-flight and how that can affect cortisol levels in the body. Well, stress also affects the gut because when you are in a high state of stress, the gut changes in response—think constipation, diarrhea, acid reflux.[138] We have found practicing meditation and mindfulness to be very beneficial for the gut.

Detoxification

Detox has become such a hot topic. And very controversial. Some detox programs take things to the extreme—like water or juice fasting, only consuming one food for an extended period, or eating and drinking weird herbal combinations. Are they really necessary?

Pam

Before we give you the answer, I'm going to share my own story. In my early fifties, I started experiencing diarrhea every day, and it came out of the blue. After visiting multiple conventional medical doctors, it was finally suggested that I have a sigmoidoscopy, which examines the lower part of the colon. It showed I had an autoimmune condition called microscopic collagenous colitis, which meant I had some pretty severe inflammation in my lower intestine. This came as a huge shock to me because I am an extremely healthy person! The conventional treatment for this disease is steroids, but there was no way I was going to take steroids, so I sought out functional health care. After doing a DNA test and an environmental toxins blood panel, I learned I was loaded with environmental toxins (think pesticides with brand names that we can't mention here), and to make matters worse, my body genetically has a difficult time naturally detoxifying itself. The good news is I have been able to heal my gut naturally by using detoxifying supplements, eating an anti-inflammatory diet, eliminating alcohol, limiting sugar intake, finding the right hormone program, and using meditation as stress relief. I was told by my GI doctor I would never be able to do this without medication, and I proved him wrong. My autoimmune colitis is in complete remission!

Us

The reality is, in the United States, you would be hard-pressed to find someone who doesn't have some environmental toxins in their body. The human body is designed to detoxify naturally, but in the twenty-first century, it just can't keep up with the toxic load. Toxins are literally in everything, and women get it the worst. Again, there are toxins in our food, plastic water bottles, perfumes, cosmetics, personal care products like shampoo, conditioner, and lotions, and even in our water supply.

The sneaky thing about toxins is that most of them are fat-soluble, which means if you don't get rid of them, they are stored in fat cells. We truly believe this is one of the reasons obesity has become such a problem in modern times. In fact, it may at least in part result from your body's protection from the adverse actions of these toxins, which, when enveloped by fat, cause us less harm.

So, to answer our earlier question about whether detoxification is really necessary, we would give a resounding yes! Many women are already struggling with excess weight from hormone imbalance, but without detoxification, it makes it harder not only to lose weight but to keep it off.

Now, we are not proponents of the starvation detox programs you may have heard of. There are many ways to safely detox while still eating real food. Many of the clients we work with tend to struggle with addictions to foods like sugar, cheese, processed foods, pizza, ice cream, and alcohol. After working with clients for over fifteen years, beyond a doubt, we have learned that sugar and cheese are two of the most addictive foods. They stimulate the same part of the brain as cocaine!

These clients are perfect candidates for a food-based cleanse, and it's something to consider if you have been feeling crappy. In our experience, clients who detox several times per year feel better, sleep better, have less brain fog, and have lots of energy. There is a cleanse program we have used for years with clients, and we have found it to be very effective for reducing cravings, increasing energy, and overall better health. In our book portal, we share our favorite products that we use to cleanse our bodies daily and quarterly. Here are some additional ways you can support your body:

Drink water: Water is life! Believe it or not, your body is around seventy percent water, and being properly hydrated is essential for optimal health. Staying hydrated is one of the easiest ways to be kind to your body and keep all systems working as they should.

Earlier, we discussed toxins a bit. We cannot stress enough the importance of drinking clean, filtered water. You might be surprised to learn the water out of your faucet is full of chemicals. Water from plastic is not good either because many plastic bottles contain a chemical that mimics estrogen (these are called xenoestrogens), which creates chaos with our hormones.[139] So if you haven't already, now is the time to invest in a good water filter or reverse osmosis system.

Drinking plenty of clean, filtered water is essential to helping your kidneys move waste through your body, which will help with moving out the toxins! The gold standard is to drink one half of your body weight in pounds in ounces of water per day.

You may not know this, but here are seven signs of dehydration:

- Fatigue
- Dizziness
- Headaches
- Bowel interruptions
- Dry skin and wrinkles

- Weight gain
- Anxiety and mood swings

Do you have a difficult time drinking enough water? Here are some tips to get in the habit of drinking more water:

- Invest in a reusable, refillable water bottle, and make sure it's made of either glass, steel, or toxin-free plastic. A quick note here: Even plastic bottles that say BPA-free plastic may still have the harmful chemicals BPF or BPS, so do your research. Get something fun that you will use and carry around with you as a reminder to drink more water!

- Set a timer on your phone to drink a few sips of water every thirty minutes until it becomes a habit, or check out the WaterMinder, Hydro Coach, or Gulps apps.

- Drink a glass of water when you first wake up and before meals. Remember, we generally wake up dehydrated. Think about it: You have been in bed for seven-plus hours, and your body would love some hydration. Rather than reaching for coffee, grab a glass of water. You will be amazed at how quickly your body wakes up.

- Flavor your water. Good choices are cucumber, orange, lemon, lime, or berries, or you can use herbs like mint, basil, or rosemary.

Eat your vegetables: Pam wrote the recipes for the cleanse we use on our website. And it's full of vegetables. While clients are initially afraid they'll go hungry, we find that is *never* the case! Instead, they say they struggle to eat all the food we give them. How could that possibly be?

When you give the body the foods it needs and wants—nutrient-dense foods—you feel full. Low-starch vegetables like broccoli, cauliflower, green beans, zucchini, fennel, tomatoes, eggplant, peppers, onions, garlic and greens give an additional detox boost.

Be mindful: Mindfulness is a practice based on Zen Buddhism. Mindful eating, quite simply, is being fully attentive to your food. And that is in all aspects of food: buying, preparing, serving, and consuming it.

In today's fast-paced world, eating has become a mindless act. We eat prepackaged or fast foods while in the car, watching TV, playing on our phones, or at our desks while working. Eating quickly, or mindlessly, tends to lead to overeating. Did you know it takes around twenty minutes for your brain to realize your stomach is full?

When you choose to eat mindfully, you are eating with no distractions and making it an intentional act instead of an automatic one. You will eat more slowly, savor your food, and give your brain a chance to catch up with your stomach.

It's not hard to get started. Here are some things you can do to eat more mindfully:

- Make a shopping list.
- Eat with an appetite, but don't wait until you are starving!
- Give appreciation to your food—believe it or not, appreciating your food can change the energy of the food![20]
- Rid yourself of outside distractions. Put down the phone and turn off the TV.
- Eat slowly, and don't rush. Take notice of what you are eating.
- Focus on how the food makes you feel.
- Stop eating before you are completely full.

When you begin to eat more mindfully, you will have more appreciation for your food and might even find new enjoyment in food. It promotes a healthier relationship with food, and you will have better nutrient absorption. By slowing down and taking the time to properly chew your food, you will also have less bloating and better digestion. In our experience, clients who have learned the practice of mindful eating have a healthier relationship with food and make better food choices.

Take Time to Feed Your Soul

PAM

For over thirty years, I've been dedicated to learning everything I can about food and nutrition, not just through reading but also through my coursework at the Institute of Integrative Nutrition. I've studied how food and nutrition affect our bodies and numerous dietary theories. I've worked with clients on their food and lifestyle choices. What was my biggest revelation? I learned that what we feed our souls is *primary* food, and what we eat is secondary.

Integrative nutrition means we view the body as a whole. While the foods we eat are certainly important to health, what we feed our soul is what sustains our life. These are the things in life that bring joy and fulfillment and make life worth living. The "nutrition" that goes beyond the plate includes healthy relationships, being creative, physical activity, a satisfying career, education, a happy home, home cooking, social connections, creative outlets, spirituality, healthy finances, and a healthy body. What you feel passionate about is probably a primary food for you.

When primary foods are balanced, your life feeds you, and what you eat is secondary. You need both for optimal health and to feel great! Think back to when you were a child, playing outside and having fun. Mom called you in for dinner, but you weren't hungry because the passion and energy of what you were doing took all your attention.

So when you are feeling off balance or lost, it is most likely an imbalance in either primary or secondary foods. If you eat too much unhealthy food, you'll feel off. When you are too stressed at work or struggling with a relationship, you'll feel off. Both situations can lead to heightened emotions or moodiness and can lead to cravings. This can be a great opportunity to dive deeper and find out what your cravings are telling you. Do you need more water? Or is your body missing nutrients? Are you craving comfort and stillness? Or could it be that you need some mental stimulation? We talk so much about how menopause is a time of transition, and now might be just the right time to discover what is feeding your soul.

We felt it was so important to include a chapter on food because diet and lifestyle play such a vital role in overall well-being and quality of life. As women, our bodies are changing so much during these midlife years. It's a good time to take an inventory of what has worked and what maybe doesn't work anymore. Honey, you can't sit around drinking wine and eating chocolates; you just won't feel your best! Our wish for you is to live with health, vitality, and joy and to honor yourself by making the best lifestyle choices possible.

CHAPTER 7

YOU ARE WORTHY

"There is something so special about a woman who dominates in a man's world. It takes a certain grace, strength, intelligence, fearlessness, and the nerve to never take no for an answer."
—Rihanna

The menopausal years can be a time when you choose to reassess your goals and priorities. Perhaps you are in an unfulfilling job or your career path isn't panning out the way you thought it would. Menopausal symptoms can play a big role in that. This is also the time of life when retirement may feel nearer—all the while, you may still have a mortgage, tuition expenses, or an aging parent's needs for support. Midlife women, in particular, face different hurdles and concerns than midlife men. While this time of life may present some unique challenges, we are going to dig in and share how to use your inner wisdom to mindfully navigate this transition.

Career

"In our third act, it may be possible to circle back to where we started and know it for the first time."
—Jane Fonda

As the population of empowered, second and third-generation career women ages, contemporary thinkers like Avivah Wittenberg-Cox have been inspired to examine what she calls the "longevity revolution" and how personal transformation over a lifetime impacts our careers.[140]

Many women in midlife find themselves at a pivotal juncture—a time of introspection and awakening, when a deeper sense of meaning and purpose in work begins to matter more. At the same time, the work landscape itself has shifted dramatically in recent years, especially since the pandemic. The old rules of success no longer apply—and that opens up exciting new possibilities. People are redesigning their jobs to accommodate work-life balance, including dialing back their work hours or working remotely. More and more people are searching for work with meaning and are choosing to forego traditional achievements like job titles or big salaries in exchange for careers that feed their souls. The truth is, many of us have inherited a narrow definition of success—one shaped by a patriarchal system that offers only a shallow vision of what's possible.

There are over forty-one million women over forty in the workforce, and on average, we will spend over twenty-four years of our working years in the menopause life stage.[141] One in every ten women will leave their jobs due to menopause-related symptoms.[142] And menopause costs American women $1.8 billion in lost working time every year.[143] Perimenopause begins when we are usually at the top of our game in our careers, requiring us to have the energy and brain power to perform well. And the symptoms of menopause can derail our professional opportunities and our futures. Not great timing.

Midlife women in the traditional workspace face obstacles, and unfortunately, employers aren't doing enough to address the issues—yet! As the menopause conversation becomes normalized, we are hopeful for change. Some women have shared feelings of shame about experiencing brain fog and not performing at their full potential. Some choose to leave their careers in search of roles that better accommodate their symptoms—while others opt out of the workforce entirely.

Besides the obvious physical symptoms, there are other reasons women may decide to make a midlife career change.

- **Fulfillment and purpose:** Women may feel they want to align their careers with their passions or values.

- **New challenges:** Yes! Some women may feel bored and ready for something new. That's not uncommon at this age.

- **Life changes:** Women who become empty nesters or who need to care for aging parents might seek different career opportunities as their priorities shift.

- **Finances:** Making any career change comes with financial considerations, and in midlife, some women may be reassessing their financial futures.

- **Work-life balance:** As mentioned earlier, more and more employees are seeking better work-life balance.

Are you ready for a career upgrade? Are you longing for something different but feel you're not quite up for it? According to a *Forbes* article by Judy Schoenberg and Linda Lautenberg, women reaching fifty have the following fears regarding their careers:[144]

- Is it too late?
- What do I have to offer?
- Am I too old?
- Will my skills be relevant?
- Will I be perceived as unable to keep up with the latest technology?

The decision to pivot careers in midlife is truly an act of courage. You are declaring you are not bound by your past but are driven by the vision of what your future may hold. By embracing the unknown, you might just uncover your true self. Now, is this easy? You may have doubts, you may worry about ageism, or you may fear the uncharted waters of a new career. These are all valid, as they would be in any new experience! However, in times like these, you may discover some of your greatest strengths.

In following their dreams, their imaginations, and the memories of what they were most inspired by as younger women, many of our clients and friends are thriving in new adventures and pivoting to more fulfilling careers. And you know what that means: You can too!

We have our life-changing midlife career story: Post-pandemic, we were at an event together, and after the event, we began discussing midlife. A few days later, we met for lunch—and found out we were experiencing telepathy! Both of us were considering launching some kind of program to support women in midlife, and Julie asked a lot of questions about Pam's sex life, but that's a story for our podcast! We decided women *need* to know what we know. So we launched our Midlife Upgrade business. Both of us are qualified for many different careers, but we felt called to build this movement to support midlife women.

We have a very generous and creative friend, Teri Turner (@nocrumbsleft on Instagram) who has always loved food. And she was known for trying new recipes and delivering the goodies to her friends and neighbors. If someone was ill or their kid broke an arm, she was in the kitchen whipping something up to brighten their day and feed their tummies with delicious food. And every single time we ran into her, it was at a wonderful coffee shop or a fun restaurant.

She was a "foodie" before there were foodies! After fully launching her children, our longtime friend (who'd gone through a divorce when her kids were in grade school) was up for a new challenge. Beginning with an Instagram account of only forty-four people who enjoyed her food photos and recipes galore, she cultivated new followers by engaging very openly with them and began creating an amazing community of food lovers. She was then approached by an online magazine, and after writing several food blogs, she noticed her numbers started growing. Her account is always joyful and promotes healthy, delicious food, too.

She now has nearly half a million followers on Instagram and another half million on other social media platforms. In addition to posting recipes, writing a fantastic cookbook, and interviewing friends, family, chefs, and culturally interesting people for her podcast—which came about unexpectedly when she interviewed her queer kid and it went viral—she also posts travel stories.

Teri's is a tale of doing what she's always loved, but now for a virtual audience of a million viewers. As part of this upgrade, she's also become a swimsuit model at the age of sixty! "You don't need the perfect body to enjoy wearing a swimsuit!" she proclaims happily. Now that is a fabulous midlife upgrade!

Looking to spend more time doing what she loved, a friend retired early from her corporate law career to open a yoga studio—trading intensity for a fulfilling and successful venture that resonates across generations. She has created a curriculum for public schools, and her yoga instructors volunteer, offering free yoga classes for the students and faculty. She feels incredibly satisfied and loves contributing to the wellness of her community.

Yet another friend accepted an early retirement package from her longtime employer in the beauty industry and is now gloriously immersed in pottery. She invests her time as a ceramist in an art form that doubles as meditation, creating unique pieces that sell enthusiastically at galleries and online. She supports herself entirely through sales of her beautiful ceramics, while occasionally lending her marketing expertise to beauty brands that seek her out. She is thoroughly enjoying this vibrant third chapter of her life.

When guiding our clients through major career decisions and practical next steps, stories like these remind them of unique gifts and talents they may have set aside decades ago. These examples reawaken possibilities and illuminate paths they hadn't considered possible at midlife.

We offer a meditation here for you to enjoy. The audio is available in the book portal. Click on the **QR Code at the beginning or end of our book.**

Set a timer for ten minutes and sit in silence for a moment; allow your mind to relax and see what comes up. Consider journaling your thoughts.

- What are your hobbies?
- What are some of your unique talents?
- What are your heart's desires?
- How did you spend your most joyful times?
- What gives you pleasure, makes you feel free, and motivates you?
- Was there a second major you considered in college or a career path you rejected because these were impractical?
- If money were no object, what would you pursue?

Once you have a vision, open yourself to transformation without even knowing how you'll get there.

Money

"Nothing could be more destined, natural, and right than women wielding wealth."
—Kasia Urbaniak

How often do you discuss your finances with your friends? We are both very open about most things, but it's not often that we discuss money with even our closest girlfriends. If we want to change our lives and change the world, we have to talk about the important stuff. And we know one thing with absolute certainty: Our world will be a much better place when more women have genuine opportunities for financial security and abundance!

Here's the current unfortunate situation. During the pandemic in 2020, women around the world lost more than $800 billion in income, equivalent to more than the combined GDP of ninety-eight countries![145] And that estimate doesn't even include wages lost by women working in the informal economy: low-paid sectors such as domestic workers, garment workers, and food-service workers. Even before the pandemic, women and girls put in 12.5 billion hours of unpaid work every day.[146] In 2021, an additional forty-seven million women worldwide were expected to fall into extreme poverty, living on less than $1.90 a day.[147] According to the World Economic Forum, closing the global gender gap has increased by a generation from 99.5 years to 135.6 years due to negative outcomes for women in 2020."[148] Yes, this news sucks.

In the United States, women sixty-five and older are twice as likely as men of the same age to be living in poverty, and that is due to women, of course, spending more of their time on free labor.[149] *The New York Times* estimates that if American women earned minimum wage for the unpaid work they do around the house and caring for relatives, they would have made $1.5 trillion just in 2019, and globally, that number was $10.9 trillion.[150] Let's face facts. Would men do that much s**t for free?

Julie

I remember hearing Suze Orman, author of *Women and Money*, speak about free labor a couple of decades ago when my son was just a toddler. She shared the salary a typical woman in the United States would be earning if she were being paid for all the jobs she did for her family. It was the first time I had even considered that I should be compensated for all of the hours that I was logging as a mother: being a chauffeur, babysitter, chef, tutor, housekeeper, etc. I really should have been earning close to $300,000 a year when I added it all up. Having children is the biggest predictor that a woman will go bankrupt in her lifetime.[151] For heterosexual couples, a mother's workload increases by 8.5 more hours per week than a father's.[152] This doubled during the pandemic.[153]

I had a very successful career before becoming a mother and choosing to parent my son full-time. I loved being a mother, which was a surprise to me because for as long as I can remember, I thought I would never have kids. It was a joy to spend my days in the company of this fun little human. But I hadn't realized that I would lose out on ten years of income, as well as retirement and Social Security benefits. I figured my husband and I would be married forever, and I would recoup the lost income when I returned to work. That wasn't exactly how life played out.

Even in the most equitable of divorces, in all of my research and my conversations with clients and friends, women don't often seem to make out with the money bag. Often, they don't receive financial equity commensurate with the work they invested into those decades of their lives. With "gray" midlife divorce, women experience a 45% decline in their standard of living, and 27% of all women will fall into poverty post-divorce.[154] Triple the rate of men.

One of my dear friends created a thriving business with her then-husband. It was super successful and profitable. He was a European citizen and told her it was in their best interest to make all deposits from the business into an offshore bank account. She loved him, was busy building their business, and was the primary caregiver for their daughter. He was managing the finances. Sound familiar? He essentially hid the business income in the offshore account. When he filed for divorce, he showed no income, so she got no spousal support. She is an extraordinary woman doing her best to create financial solvency. I am certain that I am not the only one who has held the hands of friends with stories like this.

Pam and I don't think any woman can ever have enough financial security. We may be financially vulnerable at some point in our lives, and for many of us, for most of our lives. In a society where we don't have equitable rights, even those of us who are financially solvent can find our fortunes changing in an instant. Far too many women realize in midlife that they have been providing for everyone but themselves.

One evening last summer, I attended a financial planning event for women and had an enlightening conversation with a very well-known woman in finance. "Suzanne" is considered to be one of the most powerful women on Wall Street. Like so many women who face challenging life events, Suzanne decided to use her experience to benefit others. She created an investment firm dedicated to supporting and serving women.

I was moved and shocked by our conversation. Suzanne shared with me that in her first marriage, she and her husband were both successful finance professionals, and she had a higher income than he did. Her financial success was a factor that contributed to his affair and their subsequent divorce. And even though she was earning more money than he was and had her MBA, she let her husband manage the finances. I got the impression that the divorce was challenging and didn't work in her favor. One might assume this brilliant and powerful woman, uber-successful in an industry primarily dominated by men, would have made awesome decisions that supported her financial well-being. Unfortunately, it didn't roll that way.

In Suzanne's second marriage, her husband was earning more than she was when they married. She didn't like the idea of discussing divorce before the marriage and decided against a prenuptial agreement. I've heard this before. Now, she has a very high net worth. Suzanne was super open with me and very clear that opting out of the prenup was *not* a good decision. From our conversation, it seemed she was leaning toward divorce again but delaying it, knowing she would have to give millions to her spouse. Even though Suzanne is an extremely successful and savvy businesswoman, she made decisions that harmed her financially. Her generous honesty helped me release some of the shame and sadness surrounding my own disempowered choices—choices that left me financially vulnerable after my divorce.

Oh sure, I could blame systemic patriarchy. The Wall Street powerhouse could have done the same. But our blame is not going to change our circumstances. Instead, both of us chose to transform our "mistakes." Suzanne continues to build an outstanding billion-dollar business that supports women in creating wealth and legacy. Women are alchemists, after all! As my beautiful mother says, "There has got to be gold in that pile of s**t!"

And while searching for gold, I read *The Science of Getting Rich for Women* by Sara Connell—a reinvention of a classic book from the early 1900s, that was intended primarily for men. She reveals powerful insights to help women unlock their wealth potential, offering practical, enjoyable tools to break through glass ceilings, decode the path to abundance, and overcome any upper-limit fears that may be holding us back.

Her book is a must-read for every woman. Educating yourself can also support the women in your life. She shares, "You having more creates more for others. We're not going for 'more' merely for some American, capitalistic endeavor. *The Science of Getting Rich for Women* is about authenticity, you living as big and powerfully as you desire to live. It's about you being all you came here to be, owning your absolute worth and power, whatever that means to you."[155]

There are many exercises in the book that shifted my perspective on money, helped heal feelings of unworthiness, and strengthened my ability to create wealth and abundance on all levels. Sara recommends an easy-to-accomplish morning practice that has become a very beneficial habit for me. Every morning, before I put my feet on the floor, I take some deep breaths and outstretch my arms. I simply state this mantra several times with all my heart and feelings of positive intention: "I am one with the infinite abundance of the universe." It's a delicious way to begin my day.

I'm also using my reticular activating system to focus more on the gifts of abundance and love in my life. The RAS is a bundle of nerves at our brainstem that filters out unnecessary information to allow the important stuff to get through. The RAS is perhaps in effect when you are imagining your dream vacation. You are thinking about how it would feel to be there. Wouldn't you know it: You open a magazine, and there is a photo of your fantasy destination. Of course, Instagram's algorithm is reading your mind, and there is your fantastic location yet again in someone's post. Your RAS takes what you are focusing on and then filters your experiences to show what's important to you. It's like a synchronicity machine.

Every day, I use my RAS to direct my attention and focus on noticing the gifts of abundance popping up around me. It has been like a game to look for the signs. The other day at the ATM at my local health food store, somebody had written on the machine in huge letters, "Do you love money?" And I said out loud, "Yes! Yes, I do." When I experience these winks from the universe, I feel like I'm in the flow of life. Sara Connell invites us to immerse ourselves in abundance consciousness and elevate our lives in mind, body, and spirit.

I have chosen to work with a wonderful team of compassionate and savvy women. My bookkeeper, accountant, and lawyer are all women. They have seen it all, and women advisors are more likely to understand women. After speaking with many clients and friends, our shared experience has been that male advisors don't truly *get* what stresses us out and keeps us up at night, and they are frequently unable to have true empathy for our concerns. They may not understand that being a woman means we are often behind the eight ball and that, historically, we haven't had access to the financial resources and security that men have. One fact that all of us may not know: Before the Equal Credit Opportunity Act of 1974 was signed into law, a bank could refuse a credit card to an unmarried woman, and if married, her husband was required to co-sign.

For many years, my former husband and I shared a male accountant and male financial advisors. I had created a wonderful business that supported women's health and wellness, and it was very financially successful. When I was in the early building stages, I decided to share the business with my husband, and it was set up as part of his corporation. Several years later, as my business was generating a healthy income, he was receiving payroll and retirement savings from it, but I wasn't. My income was supporting our family and his business, but not my future.

Our accountant and advisors *never* once said, "Julie, I know you were a stay-at-home mom for nine years, and then for the past few years, your business has been very profitable and is helping to support your husband's corporation. You have not had Social Security or retirement contributions for many years! Let's discuss how we can help you now make decisions to prepare for your future."

Oh that kind of guidance would have been beyond life-saving, and definitely would have helped me prepare for a possible uncertain future. And yes, I understand it was my responsibility to stay awake and take care of my finances. However, I hired a team who was supposed to be more knowledgeable than we were and support *both* of us—but they truly didn't consider how to best support me. I can only assume they figured that my husband was my security! Unfortunately, I never thought we would get divorced, and I never even considered that my retirement income would be impacted.

As I was moving toward divorce, my female attorney asked me about my assets and retirement. And that is when it hit me. I immediately called our accountant and asked him about my social security and more. His answer was, "Don't worry about social security. You are entitled to fifty percent of your husband's benefits since you were married over ten years." I fired him on the spot, and found an incredible woman to replace him.

Pam

When my husband passed away, I discovered he left me and my young daughter broke. Literally. I was an MBA and a successful businesswoman who had started multiple companies, but I blindly surrendered all financial decisions to him. He had gambled our future away in the stock market, and when he passed, he left me with over $400,000 of debt. That was a rough period in my life and a tough lesson to learn. At age forty-two, I was in the position of starting from ground zero—as a single mom. Everything I had saved for my future and my daughter's education was gone. After his passing, I also found out my husband had drained equity from our home, leaving me with a mortgage payment I could barely afford. I couldn't believe I had let myself fall into this position. I was raised to work and make sure I could always take care of myself, and I thought I had done that. But I wasn't mindful of my financial situation.

I ended up selling my home and using the little equity I had left to make a fresh start. I used that money to start another company that would give me the income and freedom I needed to raise my daughter as a single mother. It took years, but I dug myself out of debt because I knew as a single mom I had to maintain a good credit score. I am now completely in charge of my finances.

Us

We both know there are millions and millions of women having experiences similar to ours—and that many are even more disturbing. We need to learn to take care of ourselves *first*. And that doesn't come naturally for most of us. You must take a deep look at your beliefs about your worth and your family story about money and get very real about your finances and your future. Midlife is an opportunity to look at your money mindset. If you aren't in a good place with your finances, now is the time for a transformation. Maybe all you need are some tweaks.

Both of us have written short affirmations about our relationships with money, abundance, and generosity and the visions we have for our financial futures. We read them every day and have them on our vision boards. Our focus and attention are on creating an upgraded and joyful relationship with financial abundance. We encourage you to come up with some affirmations that resonate with you. And don't be afraid to ask for what you want! We are all worthy of abundance. Here are some affirmations to get you started:

- I hold the power to upgrade my beliefs.
- I am a money magnet.
- I always have more than enough money.
- I am open to receiving unlimited prosperity.
- I am worthy of financial success.
- I love money. Money loves me.

We have learned to honor our relationships with money and treat it with the love and respect it deserves. A few fun things that both of us do: We have both written large checks to ourselves and posted them on our vision boards. We have cool passwords for our bank accounts that affirm that we love wealth. We have many million-dollar bills that we carry in our wallets.

When you have cash, keep your bills neat and in order in your wallet. When paying your bills, express your gratitude for your abundance. When you are loving up your money, it will love you back!

You can also take steps to begin building a team of people who will be your advocates! There are wonderful women out there who will be happy to support you. Don't be like us; we learned on the job!

These are some questions to ask your support team:

- I didn't get a prenuptial agreement. What can I do to protect myself now?
- I'm getting married. I'm not sure I want a prenup. How can I protect my finances and assets?
- I am a stay-at-home mom. What should I be doing financially to protect my future?
- How can I be compensated for my unpaid labor?
- When should I claim Social Security? Are there Social Security advisors? (Yes, there are.)
- How can I protect my retirement while also providing for my loved ones?
- How can I make sure I don't outlive my money?
- How do I protect my 401K and IRA if I choose to be married or am in a long-term partnership?
- Should I merge my finances with my partner or spouse? We have joint bank accounts. What happens if my partner dies or we divorce? What happens if my partner decides to withdraw all of our money without my consent? (This happened to a friend of ours who was a big-time commercial banker. Unreal *and* ironic.)
- What are the benefits and drawbacks of filing our tax returns singly or jointly? This is a big one.
- My partner/spouse and I own a house. The mortgage is in my name, but I just discovered I am not on the title. How can I amend that?

- There's been a change in my family dynamics (birth, death, divorce, etc.). Should I update my estate plans, get more life insurance, or take any other steps? What are revocable and irrevocable trusts?

- I'm planning a large expense. What options should I consider regarding handling the expense?

- I have my own business. How do I protect myself professionally and personally?

Lifelong learning is necessary for financial literacy. These are the steps we must take to prepare ourselves:

- Read personal finance books and blogs.

- Follow financial advisors on social media. We love @your.richbff on Instagram.

- Check and build your credit. Have credit cards that offer great benefits, points, etc.

- Know your credit score.

- Protect your identity online and register with the Social Security Administration.

- Be debt-free. Have an emergency fund along with appropriate retirement savings.

- Track your spending.

- Work with an accountant who can advise *you* on filing status. Decide on what is best regarding filing jointly versus single and claiming dependents if you have children.

- *Always* review your tax returns—especially if they are joint returns!

🍃 Donna's Story

As I sit writing for this chapter, I struggle. I struggle because I'm a fifty-year-old mother of six children aged fourteen to twenty-two, and I'm trying to raise them as good little humans so that they can make change and progress in our world. I struggle because I'm a business owner of a mission-based financial planning practice for families in transition established in 2020 amid the pandemic. The business is flourishing in its fourth year and is requiring more time and focus so that we can build a team and standard operating procedures and serve our clients well. I struggle because I adore my new husband and have no time to pamper him; the feelings of guilt are overwhelming. I struggle because all of this is going on while I'm experiencing some of the symptoms of perimenopause. I find hope in the pages of this chapter because it shares candid honesty, direction, and guidance that is needed. I feel I'm among friends with the readers of this book.

So, my new friends, how can I add value to your lives? Here goes. First, I'll share a little backstory because I believe you can teach best from what you have experienced, which is why I am a big fan of Julie and Pam's authorship. Like so many women, I was educated, savvy, and smart. Having been raised in the '80s, I knew the world was my oyster because the generation before me fought for my freedom in education, finances, and voice. I had a beautiful young family, an MBA, and a growing career, which, like many working moms, I gave up to follow my husband's career that took us to living abroad. Fast-forward seven years when we came back stateside, and he suddenly passed away. Fast-forward four years, and I knew I had to go back to work to support my family, but I would be damned if I didn't do it with a career change that fueled my soul and provided value to the families of this good earth. Fast-forward six years from that point, and I am an author, business owner, sandwich-generation navigator, grief worker, and mother to an amazing blended family. Whew.

What lessons have I learned that I want to share with you, my new friends? Here are a few:

- Take control of your finances. Know exactly where you stand with your assets and liabilities at this moment in time. Discuss your finances with your partner/spouse, accountant, financial advisor, and business coach. The smaller details of the bookkeeping and taxes might drive you nuts, and that is okay—find the "who" that can do it for you.

- Have an emergency/cash reserve fund of three to six months of funds to cover what it takes you to be you! We make better decisions during times of stress and grief if we know that the immediate needs for our money are covered. Give yourself this grace.

- Have plans in place for immediate, transitional, and long-term goals in life. I like to call them "need-to," "have-to," and "want-to" goals. Write them down, my friends, and look at them often.

- Plan on saving for retirement while living life to the fullest. It takes intention to do this. I am an optimist who worries. I want the years we live, from our forties and fifties until our nineties, to be full of soul expansion, abundant life, and growth experiences. To do this, you have to have a plan, set savings goals, and set spending boundaries that align with your "need-to," "have-to," and "want-to" goals.

- Focus on protection planning for your family. Discuss appropriate life insurance, short-term and long-term disability coverage, liability insurance, small business coverage, long-term care, etc., with your financial professionals. These are also topics that should be talked about in your relationships, whether with a partner or adult children. How are you protecting yourself, your family, and your/their future needs for care? How is your family protecting you? Estate documents are a *must*: will, power of attorney, and health care directive documents. The mommy in me begs you to get this done.

My new friends, I hope this information has been helpful. When I remarried in 2022, we took the time to lay our finances "on the table," update life insurance coverage and title assets, create a prenup, agree on future money strategies, and respect one another in knowing there were going to be more bumps in the road, but that we would navigate them together and be open and clear. We also agreed to have systems and outside professionals in place as a double-check for the transparency needed to protect all we are doing to support this second career, second marriage, and unlimited opportunity in life. The struggle is real, and so are the rewards. With growth is change and prosperity.

—Donna Kendrick, CFP, CDFA

Us

The more of us who choose to upgrade our financial futures, the safer and healthier our world will be for all women and humans. Madeleine Albright, former secretary of state, has shared in a public speech that supporting women and girls around the globe is a matter of U.S. national security.[156] Microloans that have been given to women have been proven to lift their entire communities.[157] (She has shared that often, microloans given to men, if not properly monitored, are spent on alcohol, narcotics, and sex.) Studies have demonstrated that women investors outperform men because they develop a plan (a money roadmap), they invest consistently, and they take a long-term approach.[158]

There is some good news on the horizon. It is estimated that by 2028, women will account for 75% of all discretionary spending.[159] Further data suggests that women are now earning the same or more than their male partners, and within twenty to thirty years, there will be a great wealth transfer, and women will be holding the purse strings.[160] We are looking forward to being at that celebration!

Regardless of where you are right now, let's remember you more than likely have some hard-won wisdom. With planning, courage, and determination, you have the power to discover meaningful and fulfilling work and take control of your financial future—things aren't over yet! Let's not sugarcoat this. Fears will creep in, as they do when we decide to take charge of our lives and make a shift. Let go of any limiting beliefs, and trust that your best next chapter is still being written. Our wish is what we have shared empowers you to take full control of your choices so that your best life starts *now*.

Here is the final golden nugget from this chapter: Let Kasia Urbaniak's words from *Unbound: A Woman's Guide to Power* resonate through your entire being: "Claiming and wielding wealth is a woman's birthright. NOW IS YOUR TIME TO CLAIM IT."

CHAPTER 8

WHEN GRIEF ARRIVES MIDJOURNEY

"Grief can be the garden of compassion. If you keep your heart open through everything, your pain can become your greatest ally in your life's search for love and wisdom."
—RUMI

"Sometimes I sit and cry alone. Why is everything so hard? I try and hold everything together but honestly, I'm just exhausted."
—FROM A MENOPAUSE SUPPORT GROUP

How much time do I have left? Have I done all I can?
I wish I'd known how hot I was in my twenties.
Why didn't I freeze my eggs?
Sex hurts. Will I ever feel sexual again?
I am unhappy in my marriage.
I have lost touch with a lot of my friends.
My children are gone, and the house feels so empty.
I'm an orphan; both of my parents are gone.
Everyone's retiring, and I still don't know my purpose.
Someone called me ma'am. Seriously?
I hate that I'm supposed to check the box that says widow.
I cannot even remember the last time I was hit on.

If you have made it to midlife, you have experienced grief. Research shows that by the time women hit age fifty, over half have experienced many massive life-changing events—anything from empty nesting, divorce, mourning a major loss, teenagers failing to thrive, adult children failing to launch, caring for aging parents, death of parents, health scares, career shifts and for some women, and just the idea of turning fifty can be a life-changing event.[161] This is even before we toss into the mix the chaos of menopause.

Pam has lived through the death of her first husband, the death of family members and dear friends, the loss of friendships and pets, and a miscarriage. Julie has lived through the loss of a marriage, the death of her beloved aunt and uncle, who were like parents, and the death of one of her best friends. We have both lived through the loss of relationships—romantic ones and friendships. We grieve not following some of our dreams and wonder about missed opportunities. We have struggled with serious health issues and sometimes grieve our former thirty-year-old bodies.

Often in our culture, grief is seen as a taboo subject (much like menopause, eh?). We don't want to be perceived as weak or depressed. We are uncomfortable sharing our deepest feelings and our "sad stories." However, when we explored with women what they were struggling with in midlife, we uncovered that many women were experiencing grief, and we learned grief was a common theme in the midlife years. This is a time of great transition and change, not to mention that the mood swings that go along with midlife can magnify the feelings of grief.

It's almost as if midlife opens the portal for all the unsaid, undone, and unresolved, and the road that lies ahead may feel unpredictable, lonely, and even frightening. We found very little supportive information on midlife grief while doing research for this book; therefore, we decided it was essential to address this topic. Grief plays an integral role in the emotional down-and-dirty of midlife.

What happens in the midlife years? It can be a destabilizing time with our career: Our position may be plateauing; we may be searching for a deeper sense of purpose or possibly considering retirement. Some women have chosen to abandon jobs they love due to debilitating menopause symptoms. Women may experience feelings of emptiness or loss of purpose. Some women feel like their bodies are betraying them. Many women in midlife experience health challenges. Relationships with our loved ones and friends might shift. Children are growing up and leaving home. There might be struggles in caring for aging spouses or parents. There might be divorces and death. Maybe there are regrets. We stuff it all down and push on until midlife hits—and there they are, the unattended sorrows lurking in the background, waiting to be addressed.

Multiple losses can be overwhelming. We might lose a parent while going through divorce, a career setback, or the death of a sibling or friend. Some women are caught in the middle of raising children *and* caring for aging parents—or preparing for empty nesting *and* reckoning with the mortality of their parents. You may feel like you don't have the time or the energy to process or grieve each loss fully, which can lead to emotional detachment or debilitating numbness. In her wonderful book, *Grown Woman Talk*, Dr. Sharon Malone says, "Grief can be uncontrollable and difficult to diagnose—especially as we get older and experience compounding losses, sometimes at an alarming rate. And unlike other types of recovery, which breed resiliency, we don't necessarily get better at grieving the more we experience it. Every loss is unique."[162]

In interviewing midlife women, one of the themes that kept coming up for us was also loss experienced during the pandemic: loss of a sense of purpose, loss of friendships, loss of economic stability, loss of sending kids off to school, loss of time spent with friends and even strangers, loss of connection. Some women said they felt like they lost their sense of self!

We want to discuss the impact of the pandemic because almost every woman we interviewed for this book mentioned how it created huge shifts and losses in their lives. It seems that the pandemic magnified grief for a lot of women. It's not something we seem to be comfortable talking about; perhaps we want to forget that it even happened. Yet, it puts grief at the forefront of our consciousness. There was the obvious loss of life being constantly reported, but also, with disruptions in daily routines and significant changes to "normal" life, grief became a collective experience. There were losses of graduations, weddings, holidays—even basic events like family dinners or gatherings.

Women especially felt a loss of their support systems due to physical distancing, and the virtual connections just didn't seem to cut it. Psychologist Shelley E. Taylor, PhD, has presented an interesting lecture on how women and men cope differently with environmental stress. While men might choose the traditional "flight-or-fight" response, she presented that women "tend and befriend."[163] What this means is that during times of high stress, women "tend" to their children and "befriend" by gaining support through social networks. It makes sense, as women were traditionally the caretakers of children. During the pandemic, there was a lot of fear, anxiety, uncertainty, and the loss of the connections that offered us a sense of joy. The most important issue that women shared with us was about the loss of community and friendships because of isolation or political beliefs.

Women have been generous enough to share their stories with us. Pam posed a question about grief in a menopause group on Facebook that received a very large response. She asked, "Are any of you struggling with grief?" and was surprised by the responses. Women said things like "I don't have anyone to talk to about it" or "I don't want to seem like a complainer." "My brother died years ago, and I still struggle with that." "I cry all alone all the time." "My grief seems magnified during menopause." "I'm a single mom, and my kids are off at school. My friends are happy their kids are gone, but I feel so empty and alone." Some women shared that they cry frequently, without warning and without understanding exactly why. And then they feel like they cannot share their tears because others may not relate to them.

We feel it's important to dispel some of the myths surrounding midlife. One of the most common misperceptions is that midlife is a time of crisis—upheaval and turmoil that must be addressed with great care and caution. While midlife years can bring about significant change and transition, many women report feeling happier and more satisfied with their lives during this period as they move through these changes. For some women, it's necessary to go through very challenging times to get to the other side.

If you are ready to move through and embrace grief, it's good to remember that midlife is a time of powerful transition. Like with any transition, there are bound to be shifts. Women may question the assumptions and beliefs that have led them to this point and may begin exploring their next chapter. While this transition can be challenging, it can also be liberating and transformative if you let it. Midlife grief is part of the human experience, and it is an opportunity to discover new aspects of yourself and a life that might be more beautiful than you've ever imagined. In public interviews, Eleanor Mills, the founder of the Noon midlife community, shares a woman's story: "I went through so much, I shed so much, my marriage, my parents, the job that had defined me, but now I am 55, and I have never been happier, I've got my life set up just the way I like it."

Hormonal changes during this time may exacerbate the grieving process. You already know about the mood swings, hot flashes, and other physical symptoms—these can worsen the emotional impact of grief. Grief can be very sneaky. It can be a sound, a smell, or a song, and the next thing you know, there are tears. There is no one way to grieve and no right way to grieve. Everyone's experience will be different. And that's ok! Some days, you might feel angry. Other days, you might feel numb. And some days, you might feel overwhelming sadness and want to spend the day in bed sobbing. Allow yourself to feel full of whatever comes up without judging the feelings or trying to fix them.

Let's talk about some of the bigger losses women experience in midlife that can trigger feelings of grief.

Death of Parents

While losing a parent at any age is difficult, this can be one of the most significant losses in midlife. In the paper "Reactions to the Death of a Parent in Midlife," authors Barbara Sharlach and Jill Fredricksen write, "Coping with the death of one's parents has become a normative developmental task of midlife. Between the ages of forty and sixty, more than 50% of American women will experience the death of one or both parents."[164] As parents age and pass away, you may be left to deal with feelings of loss and grief and a sense of your mortality. It can be an extremely difficult and emotionally challenging experience, as it may also involve dealing with fear and uncertainty about the future.

In addition to dealing with loss, you may also have stressors in your life, such as caring for your children and their grief and managing your career and financial concerns. Not to mention family dynamics like family drama, former relationships, and disharmony that can come up around a parent's death. There might be issues about the estate—who gets mom's jewelry, who handles the house contents—and family dysfunction and sibling issues might also be magnified.

PAM

As someone who has experienced the loss of a parent, I can attest that there are very complex emotions that can go along with this experience. Watching my father suffer from congestive heart failure was gut-wrenching, and seeing him go through hospice care was a reminder of his mortality. And my own. My father was once a big, strong, hard-working man, and I watched him become more and more debilitated through his illness. He was a fighter, though: Given only weeks to live, he gave us ten months.

I vividly remember him in his room in hospice care and seeing that all he had left in his possession was his phone. He was wearing a hospital gown. His wallet was with my mom. All the material things he had worked his whole life for didn't matter anymore. The finality of it all struck me. Hard. While I was grateful that I had the time to spend with him while he was sick, it slowly began to sink in that he would miss my daughter's high school and college graduations, seeing me get married again, and even seeing any possible great-grandchildren. I still grieve that he won't know the amazing woman my daughter has become.

When he finally passed, it was bittersweet. Despite knowing what the outcome would be, I was still completely unprepared for his actual passing. On the one hand, it was a blessing he was no longer in pain and suffering, but on the other hand, the reality of him no longer being there hit me hard. In the aftermath of his passing, I found myself questioning whether I had done and said everything to show my love and appreciation for him. I still grieve him and think of him often—and I miss his witty, dry humor. Losing a parent feels like the end of an era.

JULIE

In the fall of 2022, I had back-to-back losses. My divorce was finalized in September. At the end of October, my aunt told me she was taking more naps and didn't feel her usual perky self. I was always in close contact with her, as she was like a mother to me, having had no children of her own. She had been coughing sometimes on our phone calls, but she told me she was having a little cold and sinus issue. It felt off to me, and I urged her to check in with her doctor immediately. Unfortunately, my aunt had smoked when she was younger, and when I would visit her, she would still sneak away and smoke a few cigarettes. She was devoted to my uncle, the love of her life, who had passed away seventeen years earlier. And she was living alone, having never fully recovered from the heartbreak of his loss.

In November, I received a call from her close friend, who shared with me that my aunt was coughing up blood. I absolutely could not imagine the worst. I immediately flew down to South Carolina to be with her. The morning after I arrived, she was taken to the hospital. We found out that she had lung cancer with multiple tumors. She was very fortunate that she could afford the best care, but unfortunately, it was too late.

It all happened very fast. Time accelerated painfully. All I wanted to do was to care for her, be with her, and love her. I planned to be with her throughout her entire journey until she passed. One morning, a palpable sense of peace filled her home. My aunt and I held hands, hugged, talked a little bit, and I read to her. I thought, "Let this peace be with us until she decides to pass." I expected at least another month with her and hoped for three months. The next morning, she was in the hospital, unconscious, dying. My head was next to hers, my hand was on her heart, and I whispered prayers into her ear. She passed in a few hours, with only me next to her and another friend, who was like a son to her, at her feet. I recited the rosary, which she loved, and prayed that my uncle would be waiting for her.

All of it was shocking to me. I expected my aunt to be at my son's college graduation in the spring. I couldn't believe she was gone. She *always* had my back. My goodness, I loved and missed her so much. Her death, following shortly after my divorce, cracked my heart wide open. A well of grief opened inside me and touched all of the sadness I had forgotten or buried for decades. It felt like my heart was on the outside of my body, and I mourned every day for months. And some days, living just felt far too difficult. It has been over two years, but something rather miraculous has emerged from the grief. Now, I feel softer, more open, and more loving. I smile and laugh more than I ever have. I am deeply loving and cherishing my family, friends, and the simple goodness of my life. And my aunt is with me all the time now. She still has my back . . . just in a different way.

Death of Friends or Close Relatives

By midlife, some women have either lost close friends or relatives other than a parent or spouse. These losses can be as devastating, if not more devastating, than losing a parent. Women have told us they feel guilty about deeply grieving a friend because the loss is complicated. Society doesn't necessarily recognize these losses the way it does familial losses. Our culture doesn't recognize grief much at all. We have heard stories of women leaving their jobs because they were only given three days for bereavement.

Our dear friend Jen shares the story of losing her college friend Jill:

Jill had beaten breast cancer, and she was thriving in her career. However, five years after being diagnosed as cancer-free, the cancer came back with a vengeance and metastasized to her spine. Unfortunately, Jill didn't have any family capable of caring for her. Her father had passed, her mother had complicated health issues, and her brother was intellectually disabled. So, I stepped into a role that was different from just being a good friend. It was challenging to determine what Jill needed because I didn't have the full picture, wasn't present for all of her medical appointments, and wasn't next of kin. Jill did not share with me the worst parts of her diagnosis, although based on my research, the prognosis was dire. I vividly recall she and I speaking with a counselor at the cancer center who inquired about future hospice care. Jill got angry and was in complete denial that she needed to have that conversation or plan for that possibility. It was hard to witness, and I did delicately bring up and help her do some end-of-life planning. When Jill did ultimately end up in hospice, I held my friend's hand, alone, and prayed over her as she passed. Her funeral was held when I was out of town with my children, and that made grieving more difficult because I wasn't able to participate in any of the rituals that help you deal with grief, like sorting through possessions that hold memories. I did connect with some of Jill's high school and work friends, but mostly I grieved alone. I would say the hardest part of being "just the friend" is the inability to help plan or do some of the rituals that you might do as a family member. I still miss her and think of her often.

Divorce

It's not uncommon for women to decide to leave their marriages in midlife. Lawyers have a term for this, "gray divorce." In talking with women, we learned there are several reasons why they may decide to get divorced. It's not uncommon as people age and change that they grow apart. Marriages can also be strained by major life events, such as the death of a parent or a health scare. When the kids are in college, some women begin to reevaluate their lives and relationships and end their marriages. Some women choose divorce because they desire greater happiness and fulfillment. However, even if a divorce is amicable, there may be struggles with grief. After all, it's the end of a significant relationship.

PAM

Honestly, I never liked the "till death do us part" line in the marriage vows. It seems so limited and outdated. The idea of being bound to one person for life can feel limiting, especially in a world where we are constantly growing and evolving. "Til death do us part" assumes that the love and connection people feel when they marry will never change despite the challenges and transformation that life can bring. It's not unusual or uncommon for people to just outgrow each other, and I have seen that happen for many of my friends. I found a new love in my late forties, and when we decided to marry we changed our vows to say "until we no longer grow together." It just felt more authentic and realistic.

JULIE

I love this quote from Maggie Smith, author of *You Could Make This Place Beautiful*. She writes, "I could talk about what a complete mind-f**k it is to lose the shelter of your marriage, but also how expansive the view is without the shelter, how big the sky is. . ." My former husband (wasbund, as a dear friend calls her ex) signed the final papers for our divorce on our twenty-seventh wedding anniversary. I guess you could call that perfect, and I still cried frequently. I realize now that not only was I mourning the end of our marriage, but I was mourning the end of a dream. A dream of what I thought our life would be together . . . and of what I thought *my* life would be. I was also mourning for the young woman who imagined that her visions for her marriage and her life would certainly manifest—because in many ways, they didn't. And certainly, I was also mourning the loss of my youth, knowing that at 60, I stood on the edge of an unknown life.

As more time passes, it seems I am beginning to forget the memories of the difficult times that occurred during our marriage—the arguments, unhappiness, and often very intense confusion and suffering. Now I can spend time with my former husband and feel love and forgiveness for him and myself. We have gone back in time in a way to when we first began our relationship. We are friends, maybe more like brother and sister who have spent years together. He is the father of our son, and our life together might be long. I heard a girlfriend say once, "Husbands come and go, but divorce is forever."

I am reimagining and re-creating my life with faith, hope, and determination. With each passing day, the view gets more expansive. This is a path of my own design, and I am building it with the wisdom I have gathered over my lifetime.

Loss of Close Friendships

For women, our friends mean the world to us. In the midlife years, treasured friendships from years past may slowly drift away or abruptly end. The pain of losing a close friendship may be as agonizing as the loss of a love relationship. After years of bonding, relying on them for support and guidance, and sharing our deepest thoughts and feelings, losing a dear friend can feel like a huge void. The grief can be enormous—not just from the loss of happy times but the loss of unconditional love and acceptance.

Our client, Angie, shared a painful breakup experience with her best friend since childhood, Lisa. Angie and Lisa became friends in first grade and had weathered all of life's ups and downs with each other: junior high, high school, college, marriages, the birth of their children, the death of parents, and even their children growing up and leaving home. Angie said Lisa was the one person who knew her better than anyone.

In her fifties, Angie decided to leave her unhappy career and open a boutique in her town, something she had always wanted to do. As the boutique became successful, Angie admits her friendship with Lisa felt strained. Lisa had gone through a painful divorce and was in a very unfulfilling job that she was unwilling to leave because of financial constraints. It was during this time that Lisa ghosted Angie.

Angie was devastated. She said it felt like it came out of nowhere. She had always remained committed to their friendship and had supported her friend in every way she could. She was shocked that now that she had some success, her dearest friend, her "ride or die," had checked out.

At first, Angie blamed herself and deeply grieved the loss. However, as some time passed, she realized that doing this only deepened the hurt feelings. She was wise enough to seek some support from a therapist who helped her process the grief from this loss. Angie is now able to remember the past with love and compassion for her friend and still wishes the best for her.

Although no one will ever replace your dear friend, staying focused on your future will help to fill some of the emptiness left behind. With time and healing, you may be able to see that friendships evolve and the love that you shared forever changed you.

Empty Nesting

If you have kids, this can be a significant life transition as you adjust to your child(ren) growing up and leaving the family home. You are no longer seeing your kids daily or handling their responsibilities. You may feel a sense of pride as you watch your kids leave the nest and bask a little in the liberation of being relieved of child-rearing duties, but on the other hand, many women say they feel a bit lost adjusting to a quieter and emptier home.

Women shared with us that they felt a loss of identity when their children moved out on their own or went away for school. For so many years, they were mom—and were needed all the time. We have invested our love, energy, and time over the years to raise our children, and when they leave, it makes sense that we would feel a huge void. Grief is a natural and normal response to this transition that each person will experience with different intensity and duration. However, some women find it's time to enjoy the rediscovery of themselves, pursue a long-awaited career shift, explore new interests, and finally live in a clean house!

Our client Maureen, felt despondent when her only child, a daughter, left for college. At first, she said she was super excited for her daughter to go have her college experience and was looking forward to her time being hers for the first time in years. But when she dropped her daughter off at school, she sobbed most of the drive home, alone. She realized her baby wasn't her baby anymore. She returned to an empty house. Maureen had no idea where her daughter was, who she was with, what she was doing, and if she was even safe! She had to acknowledge it was a major shift in her life and one she was not prepared for. She began to deeply grieve for time not spent and things not done, questioning if she had done all that she possibly could have to raise her daughter to be the best version of herself.

Even though this is not an experience of death, it is a powerful time for grieving. After some coaching, Maureen began to rediscover who *she* was again. She had devoted so much time to raising her daughter that she had put her goals and dreams on the back burner. This, too, is a common thing that happens in midlife. Maureen always had a passion for health and wellness and decided she would love to study and become a life coach! We were delighted she had discovered a new path for herself. She is very successful, has a renewed purpose, and supports other women with their journeys.

Grief With an Illness

Dealing with a serious diagnosis can be scary and can affect many areas of your life, whether it's something sudden, such as a heart attack or stroke, or something chronic, like cancer or an autoimmune illness. You may find yourself grieving, feeling despair, anger, worry, or maybe even shock. It can be a rollercoaster of emotions, and there's no right or wrong way to respond. These are some of the emotions clients have shared with us:

- **Frustration:** Why me? What did I do to deserve this?
- **Worry:** How am I going to move forward? How will I be able to pay for treatment? How will my life change?
- **Regret:** I wish I had made healthier choices.
- **Grief:** I miss my younger, healthier self. My body is betraying me.

- **Denial:** This is not happening to me. I refuse to accept this diagnosis.
- **Feelings of isolation:** No one can understand what I'm going through.

All these emotions are normal and welcome. It's part of the process of dealing with what is happening and has nothing to do with how you will meet the challenges that lie ahead. The important thing is to allow yourself to feel all the feelings. Seek out help as needed, and reach out for support from loved ones and family. Most likely, they want to help but don't know how to support you. Stay connected as you go through your treatment because social support during this time can support your healing. Seek out support groups either in person or online to connect with others who have walked your path.

At fifty-two, our dear client Michelle was diagnosed with multiple sclerosis (MS). It was an extreme shock to her. While she had struggled with fatigue and balance issues on and off for a while, she had no idea these were symptoms of something more serious. Her initial reaction was a complete shock, followed pretty quickly by complete denial. Michelle could not believe she had MS. There was no family history, and she thought she had led a fairly healthy life. Michelle began to pick apart her past, wondering what mistakes she could have possibly made that caused this to happen to her. Was it too much binge drinking in college? Did she consume too much sugar? Was this karma for something she had done? Then she started to imagine what her worst-case scenarios might be—would she be wheelchair-bound? Would her family have to care for her? Was she going to lose her independence? Michelle felt betrayed by her body and longed for her younger self.

After some time, Michelle started to accept her diagnosis. She began researching and learning more about the illness. She joined a support group for people surviving and thriving with MS and learned from others who had been there. She was able to find a doctor with a treatment plan that worked for her. Michelle still struggles, and she will tell you she has good days and bad days. She would also tell you that some days, she's all in and working hard to feel better. On other days, she just feels bad for herself (which, by the way, is normal). While Michelle realizes MS is now a part of her life, she has somehow been able to find the gift in her illness. She has learned to shift her priorities and enjoy the good days.

Collective Grief

Here's one you may not have even considered, and it may be hovering in the background of your life. Collective grief can be experienced by a community, a society, and even a world. We have all had our share of this. The horrors of terrorism, mass shootings, natural disasters like hurricanes and earthquakes, the pandemic, and ongoing wars can profoundly impact our mental health, well-being, and even how we perceive ourselves within the context of the world.

Just like with any form of grief, you might have a feeling of a lack of control. We are unable to prevent it or do anything about it, and that can leave us feeling powerless and hopeless. Along with dealing with the immediate impact of a traumatic event, you may also experience anticipatory grief—knowing the event is not over and there is more sadness to come. Many of us experienced that during the pandemic. "When will it end?" "How will it end?" "Will I be ok afterward?" It's the sense of uncertainty that may leave us feeling helpless.

During times of extreme grief, we may have the opportunity to come together and publicly mourn. We experienced this after 9/11. Despite such a horrific tragedy, we came together to help each other heal. In challenging times, uniting with our communities can help us heal from our collective loss. It's also worth noting that, like any other form of grief, collective grief is still a deeply personal experience. If gathering with others doesn't feel good, it's okay to give yourself the space you need to heal and grieve privately as necessary.

One of the best ways to deal with collective grief is to limit media exposure. There's a saying in the news business: "If it bleeds, it leads." Unfortunately, the tragic events are the ones that attract the most headlines. There is a lot of good in the world, and it can be very healing and uplifting to look for it. You can practice random acts of kindness: wave a car to go in front of you in traffic, buy someone a coffee, offer compliments, hold doors open, volunteer. Even just a smile can brighten someone's life. You will be creating more peace in our world by just practicing simple, kind actions. As the Dalai Lama said, "World peace must develop from inner peace."

Youth and Physical Appearance

This was a big one that came up often when we talked with women about midlife grief. There's no denying we live in a culture that places a high value on youth and beauty, and it's difficult for many women to accept the physical changes that come with aging. We often feel pressure to maintain a youthful appearance to remain desirable because our culture places such importance on these qualities. Valerie Monroe, former beauty director at O, The Oprah Magazine, has written in her fabulous blog, "It is crucial to learn to love your face no matter how you choose to accept or confront the aging process, because you'll never be really happy with how you look unless you can see yourself uninhibited by objectification." [165]

Objectification—these pressures are everywhere in our culture. Advertising, social media, and celebrity all impact our expectations of what it means to be youthful, beautiful, and desirable. As we age, we will experience wrinkles, gray hair, and shape changes. But while these changes can be unsettling, no one gets out alive! Yes, it is understandable that we grieve our youth, as it's a shift to embrace that appearance is no longer a factor in how you are valued or perceived. But it's another wonderful opportunity to focus on what matters in life.

Here's the thing: We believe true beauty comes from the inside out. Drink water, eat healthy foods, surround yourself with people who uplift you, smile, and find things that bring you joy. We all know women who are older but radiate a beautiful, youthful spirit. Your inner glow is what will truly enhance your outer appearance.

We know a lovely older woman, Faith, who has done an admirable job at embracing aging. At sixty-three, she is a role model for all of it. Literally. She's a model. She has let her hair go gray and has the normal skin of a woman her age, but she is radiant. Sure, she does all the right stuff, like eating healthy, drinking water, and exercising, but she would be the first to tell you that once she let go of society's expectations of beauty and decided to embrace aging, her modeling career took off! Faith said the only thing that ever weighed her down was the expectations of others, and she says in her sixties, she is living her best life.

Ambiguous Grief

This is the sneaky form of grief, often overlooked. You have been going along, living your life as you always have—doing the right things, showing up on time, being there for everyone, feeling like everything is normal and hunky dory and BOOM—out of seemingly nowhere, there's a shift. You can't quite put your finger on it, because it's not as if everything is falling apart, and it's not as if you are falling apart, but something just isn't right. It's the loss with no name.

Unlike traditional grief, which follows a death or clear ending, ambiguous grief lingers in the gray areas. There's no funeral, no casseroles, no socially sanctioned mourning. You're grieving, but the world doesn't always recognize it. In fact, the person or thing you are grieving may still be very present, but emotionally or relationally absent. Or a person may be gone, but the loss is simply unresolved.

It's the collection of all the changes, all at once. A feeling of unease. No more periods. No kids in the house. A friendship that's faded away. A partner that may feel more like a roommate. The career that's become mundane and pointless. The pants that don't fit like they used to. A few more wrinkles on the face.

This is the grief where there was no clear idea when it started, and no definitive end. It's just the day you look in the mirror and think—what the hell happened? Is this it? Is this all there is? And what's supposed to happen next? Everything has somehow changed and you didn't even notice. Not until just NOW.

Ambiguous grief is the slow burn of what was the norm, but somehow isn't what it used to be. And there's no one word for mourning something that isn't quite lost, but also isn't quite there anymore.

We grieve what didn't abruptly end, but what softly slipped away. We grieve people that haven't passed. We grieve the person we used to be. We wonder about the what ifs? There is no clear 'before' or 'after.' There is a lack of closure. You may feel a bit in limbo, grieving what was but living what is.

And herein lies the opportunity. It's time for a deep breath and a pause. What do I want NOW? Who am I NOW? Bring yourself to the present. Name what it is you are feeling at this moment. This is the power of midlife, it's not what has faded from your past, but what you are finally waking up to. It's the quiet, sacred rebuild. And you get to write your own ending.

We love this quote by author and therapist Pauline Boss who says, "Closure is a myth. The goal is not closure. The goal is to learn to live with the ambiguity."[4]

Processing Grief

Maria Shriver wrote a beautiful article, "Everything Takes Time," and shared that many years ago, she was on a healing journey, and one of her friends was very concerned about her.[166] She told her friend, "I'm going to pull myself out of the darkness. I'm going to get to my open field. It may take some time, but I'll get there. I can see it and envision it. And when I envision something, I know I'll make it happen. I don't care how long it takes or how hard it is. I know I'll find my way."

Midlife grief is a complex and layered experience. For some women, it might simply feel like emptiness, or it can manifest physically as fatigue, insomnia, or weight loss or gain. To move through grief, we must find the courage to experience it as fully as we can manage. This may sometimes feel impossible, but it is essential if you want to heal more deeply and find more meaning in your life. There are many ways to move through grief, and it's an incredibly personal experience.

🍃 Barri's Story

In 1993, my mother Ellen died suddenly at fifty. Not only did this change the trajectory of my life profoundly, but it left many unanswered questions about my own menopausal health and future in the balance. There was a fan by her bedside, and hot flashes were a hot topic—but then she was gone. She had a brain aneurysm following a lifetime of off and on headaches that we chalked up to normal. I was twenty-seven.

As the eldest of two girls, Mom was my first and foremost trusted advisor. She was so forthcoming about everything from how to insert a tampon (and showed you by example!) to asking us about boyfriends and safe sex. She was comfortable in her skin—the kind of friend you could ask and tell most anything. She was modern before her time, and so was my grandma before her.

She and my father divorced when I was just ten, and I saw the bigger life she wanted for herself and what conscious uncoupling could look like. (I would heed that lesson myself down the road!) She created a job share with her best friend, also newly separated in the '70s. The local press named them the dynamic duo, as they shared a real estate job, business card, desk, and hours. One watched us while the other took floor time.

Our much too short time together on this earth taught me so very much. First, how to be a great Mom and mostly, how to share what we learn and glean with others, even in the most difficult times. Maybe it could make the journey that much easier for the next woman.

The loss of my mother led me to form The Memory Circle (TMC) and to work as a grief specialist. TMC is a place and space where we gather in groups to share a wisdom exchange and tools for grief tending. Being seen and heard in grief—both death and non-death loss—is a necessary part of processing loss. As this chapter shares, we can experience so much non-death loss at this life stage, like divorce, infidelity, empty nesting, mid-life changes, lost friendships, and lost opportunities (our old selves or the new ideals we imagined that never quite took shape).

The beauty of Circle or a like-minded support group is finding those who "get it" or someone who has "been there" to help us see a path of hope and healing ahead. My all-time ask is that we do the same for others who have helped us and pay it forward when the time presents itself.

I also lean heavily on writing in our groups. It has helped me make sense of my grief. We uncover that which may be hiding in the subconscious. From journaling to Substack, once I feel a collective consciousness bubbling like loneliness or a query I might have asked Mom if she were here, I send it out into the ether by sharing or exploring it in a notebook.

I think we gather, as is our nature, so we can feel part of a collective. A place to feel a sense of belonging over longing. A safe space where we can air our questions and concerns, feelings and foibles, free of shame or insecurity. Finding this outside of a doctor's office or therapist's sofa is a gift (and highly recommended). It is often where my members share their wishes and heart's desire for greater understanding and feel they've been served a big fat dose of "permission granted" to proceed with confidence and clarity. Some of the best medicines imagined or reimagined.

—Barri Leiner Grant,
Chief Grief Officer™, The Memory Circle

Connection

Both of us have lived through heavy grief. And what was most healing for us was spending time with our women friends who were unconditionally loving and just listened without judgment. They were our "ride or die" crew. They made us know that we would make it through; they offered us hope.

Grief, and specifically midlife grief, can be isolating and lonely, but we are not meant to go through it alone. Connection with others can be a powerful source of healing and help you feel understood, validated, and supported. Whether it's through the support of friends and family or by seeking out a support group or therapist, it's essential to acknowledge and process grief healthily.

> After our client, Cindy, lost her father, she shared, "One of the most healing experiences I had was just crying with a dear friend. It had been several months since my father's passing, and the phone calls and check-ins had stopped. My friend had also lost a parent and knew about the pain of that loss. One morning, she surprised me by bringing me breakfast and a coffee and just sat with me. She gave me the love and space I needed to grieve and quietly cared for me while I let my tears flow. It was very healing to be witnessed in my grief, and after that morning, I began to feel more peace."

Vulnerability

Vulnerability is an approach you may find helpful in moving through grief. To grieve fully, it's important to open yourself up to being vulnerable and to receiving the kindness and support of others. You can ask for help. This is often very difficult for women because many of us have learned to keep our emotions hidden and to push through our pain. Brene Brown has written beautifully about vulnerability. She shares that many of us try to protect ourselves from vulnerability by numbing our emotions, pretending to have everything under control, or attempting to be perfect. However, in doing so, we shut ourselves off from the possibility of experiencing love and connection, both of which would nourish us during times of grief. If possible, be honest about how you are feeling and what you are experiencing even when it's uncomfortable or messy. Find a safe and supportive space to share where you can be met with empathy, understanding, and support. As Brene has written, "Vulnerability is the birthplace of love, belonging, joy, courage, empathy and creativity."[167] As midlife women, we know that in our darkest moments, the love of our friends and our communities helped us to heal and find our way back to ourselves.

Pam

There was a time in my life when I was experiencing deep grief and cried frequently. I was lucky enough to belong to a wonderful parish at the time, and while I did not attend mass regularly, I found the priest at our church to be incredibly supportive, and his homilies lifted me. One Sunday, a wave of grief hit me like a ton of bricks, and the tears started flowing. A lovely young woman came out of nowhere, hugged me, and let me cry openly on her shoulder. She just held the space for me that I needed at that time, and I will never forget her. I asked her name, and she shared it was Angela. Although I never saw her again, she was a true angel to me at a time when I needed one.

Be Kind to Yourself!

We cannot emphasize this enough. As women, we can be very hard on ourselves. Self-compassion is crucial to the healing process. When grieving, it's easy to fall into self-criticism and blame. We may have regrets and think we should have said or done more or that we may have somehow caused the loss. Treat yourself to the same compassion, kindness, and understanding you would offer to a dear friend who is going through a difficult time.

One of the most significant challenges of grief for midlife women is the expectation that we must stay strong and be stoic in the face of loss. Women already tend to be viewed as the caregivers and nurturers and, in the face of grief, may feel the need to maintain the façade of strength and composure even when struggling with overwhelming emotions. This can make it that much more difficult to acknowledge and express grief, which can lead to feelings of loneliness and isolation.

Pam

After the loss of my husband, I was incredibly grateful to find a support group for grieving spouses. I had so many challenging feelings tied to that loss and initially felt very isolated and wondered if my feelings were normal. That group not only gave me a safe environment to express my grief but also validated and normalized my feelings. I found the group to be supportive, understanding, and non-judgmental, and it gave me the skills and resources I needed to move forward during that challenging time. Many grief support groups offer not only support and understanding but empathy and a sense of community.

I want to make a quick note here. After attending the group for many months, I began to notice it was all the same faces. I inquired and learned many had been in the group for **years.** While the group initially gave me the support I needed, I began to feel stronger and decided my loss would not define me. I lovingly said goodbye and expressed my gratitude to all of the people who held me when I needed it most.

Rest

It's okay to take time and just rest. If you have gone through any type of grief, it can be exhausting. It's completely normal to feel very depleted, and resting doesn't just tend to your physical needs; it is essential for your emotional, mental, and spiritual well-being as well. In a world where we are encouraged to "move forward" and "push through," taking time to rest is the opportunity to acknowledge your pain, honor your emotions, and grant yourself the time and space you need to heal.

Resting can mean different things to different people. It may be meditation or a restorative nap. It can mean seeking solace with loved ones or engaging in activities that bring your heart joy. Consider that which honors your need for restoration. Rest may be just what you need to lean into your grief and unfold your healing.

Deep rest might help you during times of grief. We have heard from clients that it's not unusual to need sleep for twelve to fourteen hours at a time. We don't talk enough about how grief takes a toll on us physically. However, it can also complicate sleep and the ability to rest. We have heard other women share they experienced anger, shock, denial, sadness, and fear over certain losses that caused insomnia. It's important to address these issues with a doctor or counselor, especially if they become chronic. Long-term sleep deprivation can cause depression, heart problems, and the inability to cope not only with your loss but with everyday activities as well.

The Power of Mindset

The way you think about and perceive your situation can have a huge impact on how you feel. If you focus exclusively on the negative aspects of your midlife grief, you might find it difficult to move forward. However, if you are willing and able to adopt a growth mindset, you can view your loss from the lens of an opportunity for transformation. Change is inevitable; learning to surrender and embrace it is essential. Letting go can be challenging, but the more you are willing to move forward, the more liberated you might feel.

Writing and journaling

Journaling is a helpful tool for grief tending. It can be a sacred space to safely navigate the complex emotions that go along with grieving. Putting pen to paper allows the heart to pour out thoughts and feelings without judgment. It's an opportunity to reflect on memories, untangle confusing thoughts, and honor what's been lost. Even writing a letter to a loved one can be healing. You can even ask them questions and journal their answers that might come to you. Your journal can be a treasured memory of the love you shared.

Gratitude

Gratitude is a powerful tool in any situation, but particularly in embracing grief. We all know expressing gratitude is one of the keys to having a fulfilling life. Even during extreme grief, there are things that we can appreciate. We can express our gratitude for the simple goodness in our lives: Our breath. The sky. Spending time in nature and being grateful for her beauty can be very healing during times of grief. It might help you shift your perspective. And as Queen Elizabeth II famously said, "Grief is the price we pay for love." The grief may remain and lighten, but the love will endure.

Reprioritize Self-Care

We have included information on self-care in Chapter Five, and it is essential during times of grief, though it may be challenging to honor even the simplest of your basic needs. Taking just a few minutes for a walk with healing music can bring peace, or maybe just brushing your teeth is all you can do. Of course, eat healthy foods, do light exercise that works for you, and rest your body, mind, and spirit.

Seek Professional Help

If the grief becomes overwhelming, please reach out for professional help. Seek support from therapists, support groups, healing practitioners, or spiritual guidance. Discover what is most healing for you.

Look for the Light

While it may be hard to see while you're in the midst of it, midlife grief can be a catalyst for growth and healing. As we age and endure painful loss and profound change, midlife is a gift—an opportunity to open your heart and reflect deeply on your priorities, values, and intentions for your life. As we may shed our former identities and reinvent ourselves, our clients and friends have expressed to us that their lives have become more meaningful and that their love relationships and friendships have become sweeter and more authentic. As we have lived long enough to know that life will bring joys and sorrows, we learn to treasure the moments of happiness and light.

Loss evolves, and the texture of it changes. We can discover the gift in our losses and know that grief is not something to get over but rather something to move through. If you allow it, the wisdom of grief can make you a stronger and wiser woman. Continue to move in the direction of your dreams and look for the sacredness in your journey.

CHAPTER 9

TOGETHER STRONGER: YOUR LOVING RELATIONSHIPS

"I define connection as the energy that exists between people when they feel seen, heard and valued; when they can give and receive without judgment; and when they derive sustenance and strength from the relationship."
—Brené Brown

By the time we have reached midlife, we have acquired enough wisdom and self-awareness to thoughtfully begin designing our third chapter. You may be wondering:

- Where are all the fabulous women I want to hang with?
- What about my relationship with my partner?
- Will I have love in my later years?
- How do I feel about dating?

In this chapter, we will explore love relationships and community through the unique perspective of the midlife woman. Armed with the tools we are about to share, you will feel prepared to manifest the vibrant, joy-filled future relationships your heart desires and longs for.

There is a great birthday card that reads, "And she gave no fucks. Not even one. And she lived happily ever after. The end." Hormonal and other physiological changes are contributing factors to not giving a fuck. As the ovaries wind down, the fuel of estrogen that used to pump into our emotion and communication circuits dissipates. We are no longer as interested in tending to others' needs as the neurotransmitter and oxytocin levels drop, too. And even the wonderful dopamine rush we once felt when talking with our friends has lessened. Progesterone drops too, and with it, the feelings of well-being that GABA once supported. These changes in our hormones affect the functioning of our brains and, therefore, our thoughts and feelings as well. Consequently for some of us, giving fewer fucks may lead us to shift our identity in midlife.

Perhaps an event or a series of events just shockingly shows up in our life and commands that we make major changes. Those shifts may be seismic and can include catalysts such as a major illness, the end of a marriage or partnerships, the death of loved ones, and possibly even the end of friendships. These shifts can be the beginning of a journey to a new life—at midlife.

Community

"Let's build community together because when women gather, magic happens!"
—SUZANNE GILBERG. MD, FACOG

We all know the importance of community. However, for midlife women, community can be a lifeline. It is a source of connection and can be a vital support for helping women navigate the challenges of midlife and their overall well-being. Women need to know they are not alone! A Harvard study found that the most significant predictor of our health at eighty is the quality of our relationships at fifty.[168] Even in his *Blue Zones* book, Dan Buettner found that the areas with the most centenarians have large numbers of people supporting each other in the community.

Sometimes it is not so easy to create a different community of friends in our midlife years. The relationships we made when we were younger while we were working, building careers, and raising kids may have become outdated. When the kids are grown and the former job is history, we may lose the common bonds we once shared. Our interests shift. For some, our perspective narrows, and for others, our view of life and its potential may expand immensely. We might be attending to a dissolving partnership or marriage or enjoying a blossoming love relationship while caring for our aging parents, launching our older kids, and not having a lot of time to nourish new or old friendships. We also might not feel fabulous or have the energy to cultivate relationships. We may have very limited bandwidth for the activities and people we no longer enjoy.

In midlife, women tend to experience a shift in priorities, and the superficial trappings of society might no longer hold the same allure. Instead, women are seeking meaningful connections that nourish their souls—friendships where they can share without fear of judgment. Before we began writing our book, we both did a deep dive and spoke with many, many women. They often expressed sadness regarding the loss of friends and a longing for more community. Here are a few of the responses they shared:

- "My relationships are very superficial. I'd like to have deeper friendships—friends that I could feel comfortable with being myself."

- "I want to feel good, and I don't want to drink all the time. A glass of wine is okay, but most of my friends just want to go out, drink, and gossip."

- "I have no one to talk to about the things women don't usually talk about. I want to have open conversations."

- "I don't have the time or energy to meet new people. And where would I meet them anyway?"

In *Grown Woman Talk*, Dr. Sharon Malone writes, "Recent studies have flipped the script on the science of relationships in ways that are both enlightening and encouraging, especially for women of a certain age, since most of us are without a partner or will end up there due to divorce or widowhood (harsh, perhaps, but true). Those of us with a community of friends will likely endure those life changes—and others—more easily."[169]

Julie

I intentionally began cultivating my relationships with women when I was in my final years of perimenopause. Having recently fully recovered from a ten-year autoimmune illness, I had more time, energy, and reserves for hanging out with people other than my son and my husband. Since I felt so much healthier, I had more to give, and I deeply wanted women to experience more happiness and well-being in their lives. I started inviting a few powerhouse women I barely knew to lunch. It took courage. I was still pretty raw. I was going way out of my comfort zone, and it was wonderful that those friendships blossomed.

I loved the idea of creating gatherings for all the new women in my life, so I decided to host events I called Underground Goddess Salons. At the first event I hosted, I invited over 100 women, and sixty-five showed up! All of the events were absolutely delightful. Usually, we met at a unique and fun location with very special speakers and great food. And they were free! Generous women donated their homes or venue spaces; all of the other goodies were donated, too. Sometimes we would raise money for a particular charity. More and more women found out about the Salons, and the list of attendees grew. It was a movement of sorts, and I could clearly see that women longed for community beyond their usual social circles.

Many times during my events, women would approach me to introduce themselves and start crying, sharing that they had been longing for connections like the women they had met at one of my Salons. My heart was so happy. At that time, I wouldn't have called it a sisterhood, but that's what it was: A safe, affirming space where women of all ages could fully be themselves and enjoy meeting other extraordinary women. Years later, when I was studying with Regena Thomashauer, she shared about the importance of sisterhood and the healing and empowering effect it can have on us. She has shared that "Sisterhood is Salvation," and it creates ripples in our lives and our world.[170]

One of my dearest friends in Chicago, Kathy Bresler, opened a beautiful, communal gathering place for women in Chicago called ALTAR Community. She shared with me that, "I created the space I was craving." Apparently, other women are craving this, too, because she opened during the height of the pandemic and has still managed to be very successful! More women today are seeking connection and community with likeminded women to network, collaborate, and thrive together. I regularly attend events at ALTAR and always meet new and interesting women who uplift my spirit.

There are many possibilities for creating new and lasting friendships. Women are changing the world, and wonderful opportunities are opening up every day. There's a really inspiring organization, Poker Power, teaching women how to play poker and supporting them to succeed in business, finance, relationships, and life. You can join online or in person. There are also online "dating" apps now, like Bumble, BFF, and Meetup groups, for meeting and networking with other women.

In the past few years, Pam and I have attended quite a few retreats and classes exclusively for women, and we have made many new friends we love. There are retreat centers, community centers, volunteer opportunities, and others where you can pursue your passions and find a thriving and supportive community that aligns with your heart and evolving values.

We are going to say it again: We live in a patriarchal world culture. This system is the soup we swim in . . . and it f**ks us up. Like Sheryl Sandberg, who revealed in *The New Yorker* magazine that she felt like a fraud all of her life, and Gayle King, who shared she often wakes up in the morning feeling fat. As women, we know this, don't we? We always remind our friends and clients to honor themselves when they receive a compliment. Instead of brushing it off or saying they got it on sale, we encourage them to confidently say, "Thank you. It's true!"

Regena has written, "When we live in a world that cannot even comprehend its inherent bigotry against women—and thus cannot step forward to honor or support the women and girls who have been devastated by it—what is the recourse?"[171] We believe the recourse is for women to reclaim our radiance and power and to live life on our terms. Midlife opens us to this possibility. Our desires are powerful. We are not what we have been indoctrinated to believe. As we elevate ourselves, we will elevate other women as well. We can stand for our sisters and celebrate them often! Recently, this has been encouraged and shared with the hashtag #hypewomen. We can challenge each other to be the best and the brightest and to release the very limiting and false beliefs that there isn't enough juicy goodness, happiness, or abundance to go around.

For a few years, I have been practicing with friends (and women I met during online courses and training sessions) some fun and simple things you can do regularly that will begin to bring more deliciousness into your life. You can do these in real life or via text or voice message. I read that one of Diane von Furstenberg's morning practices is sending a happy text to a loved one or someone she just feels like celebrating that day. She is a fan of emojis. Me too! Almost every morning, I text one of my dear friends and send them an uplifting message of love. It's a powerful woman who knows how to hold her radiance and invites the women around her to do the same! When we can see the goodness in ourselves, our cup becomes full so that we can then uplift other women.

You can also share your desires with your friends. That can be more difficult, as it means allowing someone to learn more about us. Sharing a desire for our lives can feel very intimate. It's not something we do every day. Your willingness to share and be open will allow others to do the same. An important caveat: it's essential to be discerning and intentional when sharing your highest dreams and desires with friends. The most beautiful part is that when you do, a trusted friend can support you in visualizing and manifesting them.

Pam and I share our desires regularly via text message. We celebrate each other and imagine our desires coming true. One of our favorites is: "We desire that our next book is a *New York Times* bestseller, uplifts millions around the world, is translated into multiple languages, and that we are interviewed on Dr. Kelly Casperson's amazing podcast, 'You Are Not Broken!'"

We imagine and honor success for one another, and this lifts us even higher. Set a reminder on your phone to celebrate your friends every day. That is the beginning of building a stronger community of love and support in your life! And we promise you that the more love you share with others, the more love you will receive!

And hey, if you feel these ideas are too big of a stretch, simply practice loving your current friends and the people you meet when you are out and about. Everybody could do with a smile and an extra dose of love! The love you are offering will be contagious, will flow back to you, keep you radiant, and might even bring a sexier sashay into your steps.

We feel very fortunate to have a large circle of women in our lives—creative badasses, many entrepreneurs, and women who have forged their paths and overcome too many obstacles to count. With these women holding our hands and guiding us through the dark passages of our midlife journeys, both of us are creating the lives we imagined for ourselves.

Contemplate and journal on the following questions to invite more harmony into all your relationships. Reflecting on these will also help you gain the clarity to release any relationships that no longer serve you.

- Who am I?
- What do I value?
- What brings me joy?
- Who are my people? Whom do I love? What qualities do I appreciate about them?
- What kinds of energy and connection do I truly crave?
- What are my boundaries?
- How do I care for myself and manage my relationships when I feel uncomfortable, taken advantage of, or hurt?

Loving Relationships

The beauty of this era of life is that there may be more space, time, and opportunity to focus on your love relationship. That may mean elevating it, taking it to the next level, and creating more intimacy and love. Or that may mean choosing to dissolve it, allowing more love to flow in a new relationship with *yourself*—as well as your relationships with others.

Just because you are in a committed relationship doesn't mean dating is off the table—just the opposite. Date your partner. Seriously! Dating in marriage or a committed relationship is the best way to keep the spark alive. We have coached women who feel lost in their marriages and feel like they don't even know their partner after so many years of being together. We ask, "Do you spend quality time together?" If the answer is no, we say, "Damn girl, go date your husband!" And here's the thing, if you don't want to, you may want to think about plan B.

However, if you still like and love your partner, schedule time together. It's so important to keep that connection going. You know, we thrive on the dopamine hits we get from doing and trying new things. Even hanging out and snuggling on the sofa while reading together or watching a movie can be delicious. Regular date nights encourage communication, break up the routine, and nurture connection and deeper intimacy. Upgrading your love relationship with your partner is a big-time midlife upgrade!

In the 1990s, Drs. Elaine and Arthur Aron developed a set of questions, referred to as the "36 Questions to Fall In Love." The research determined that two strangers can develop an intimate connection by asking each other increasingly personal questions.[172] Some of our favorites that we have shared in our relationships and suggested to friends and clients are:

- For what in your life do you feel most grateful?
- If you could wake up tomorrow having gained one quality or ability, what would it be?
- Tell your partner what you like about them.
- What roles do love and affection play in your life?

Asking your partner these questions may be a great way to reconnect. Questions like these are fun to ask, whether you are in a new relationship or have been with the same person for years. You might just learn something new about your partner (and even yourself!). Check out The Book of Questions, Hot Topics, and Couples Conversations cards. There are also fabulous intimacy decks out there too.

One of our friends, Annie, has been, in her words, "blissfully married" for thirty years. We wanted to know their secret sauce. She told us that she and her husband, Ben, go on weekly "play" dates, and it's always been part of their schedule. They've done super cool stuff together. It could be as simple as a dinner out, go-kart racing, cooking classes, pottery classes, wine tasting, escape room, rock climbing—you name it! They have regular vacations together and spend a lot of time just playing together. Being in their company is wonderful because they adore each other, laugh a lot, and are best friends. One of the other things she shared with us was about their fab sex life. They have sex on average three times a week! Talk about secret sauce.

For many women, as we begin to orient our lives more around what lights us up, our partnerships transform. Some dissolve, and others blossom. For some, change may not be possible. But it is fundamental for women to understand that we have the power and freedom to design a relationship to align with our heart's desires at this stage of our lives. The process of getting there may feel like climbing a mountain without a lot of gear and little oxygen. We know this. We lived it. And not everyone needs to go that route up the mountain. There may be a far gentler path for you. The journey begins with knowing that you have the power, and your desire can fuel that power.

One of our clients, Gigi, was married for almost thirty years when she finally chose to get divorced. She had been conflicted about the relationship and the possibility of ending it for ten years. We discussed the issues that concerned her, and she was very proactive in choosing to be in couples therapy with her husband and attempting always to reconcile their differences. One of the reasons she was struggling was that she believed she was a failure. She perceived having a successful marriage as an accomplishment. Her parents had divorced when she was young, and of course, she told herself that would never be her fate. She had hoped to preserve her marriage, but it was coming at a very high cost to her well-being.

At some point, she simply became indifferent. As for so many women, she was very busy absorbing herself in her work and raising her children. Her husband always worked long hours, so they began living separate lives, sleeping in separate bedrooms. It seems this gradual indifference is a common path for many couples as they age. What was once perhaps a relationship with more happiness and a deeper bond begins to wither and ultimately dies. Some of this may be due to the physiological changes that occur as women approach menopause. Shifts in estrogen occur as our estradiol (nature's baby-making hormone) decreases and our estriol (the estrogen that stimulates creative centers in our brain) increases.[3] We become more focused on our own lives. "When we reach menopause, all that we dreamed and did not do often comes to reproach us for having given ourselves away to others' expectations and needs. We often spend years doing this and then feel that the sacrifice done—it is not even appreciated," said Germaine Greer, a feminist voice of the twentieth century.

Gigi also realized that for many years, she had thought she could fix her husband. She worked tirelessly to help him build his business and supported him in manifesting what she thought was his potential! She invested her energy and time in boosting his life and was unable to meet many of her own needs and desires. Her thoughts were consumed by "saving" him, and she believed that by rescuing him, she would somehow create the life she desired. I recommended she read the holy grail of codependency material by Melody Beattie, *Codependent No More*. I read it in my late twenties, and it changed my life. She read it and told me she practically underlined the entire book!

Gigi began recognizing that she was very unhappy, though she was still undecided about ending her marriage, and started prioritizing her enjoyment. She began nourishing her dreams and making consistent daily choices to bring more pleasure into her life. She attended classes at the university in her city and met new people who shared her interests. A few years prior, she had begun a new career, so she felt financially stable. The fear and the reality of financial insecurity are the primary reasons that many women remain in unhappy marriages.

Late one night, Gigi literally felt a hand on the top of her head and then heard an inner voice say, "You are finished. You are complete." She told us it was as if her higher self had finally given her permission to end the marriage, and she knew it was the perfect time. Their divorce process moved along very quickly, and they have a very amicable relationship now. Their children are happier because their parents are happier.

One of the primary foundations of any successful relationship is excellent communication, and this can be very challenging when we are going through the transition of menopause. All of our symptoms can be overwhelming; our mood swings, poor sleep, lack of confidence, and a host of physical changes can put a strain on our partnerships.

If you haven't already, honor yourself and your relationship by sharing what is going on for you regarding perimenopause or menopause. Your partner might have no idea. We have a client who was struggling in her relationship because of her symptoms. The worst one was severe night sweats (the moodiness was another story). We encouraged her to be honest with her partner about what changes were happening so that they could continue to have a happy relationship. Here's what happened: he was super supportive and admitted he was wondering what was going on. Now they sleep with the bedroom temperature at a very cool sixty-three degrees. She sleeps in a T-shirt and panties, and he sleeps like he's about to go skiing. But he's happy and she's happy and well-rested.

Our dear colleague, Dr. Amy (name changed), is a urologist in the menopause space. She's now on the other side of menopause, but because this is her profession, her husband, David, is extremely well-educated on menopause. Here's the funny thing. One day at work, David's business partner said, "My wife is complaining she just got her period. I'm not sure what I'm supposed to say to that." David wisely asked, "Is it possible she's approaching menopause? Maybe she's a little shocked because she hadn't had her period for months, and this one came out of nowhere. You might tell her you're sorry she's not feeling so well. Ask her if she needs any support or wants to discuss the changes she's going through." Okay, could we love David anymore? Nothing better than a well-informed partner.

You might be in a loving relationship but feel it has lost some of its magic and sizzle, and now you are more like roommates. "Anytime, anywhere, where two hearts join, the world is brought a little closer to heaven."[173] We deeply believe these words from Marianne Williamson. We so enjoy being in the presence of very happy couples, and their love lights up the room. It's a delight to witness.

There are some wonderful resources out there that are available for creating and maintaining loving, nourishing, uplifting love relationships with a partner, as well as those that support the completion of a loveless or difficult partnership. The practices we are sharing below are useful for elevating *all* of our relationships. These are relatively easy to implement into your life and will help you to have more caring and authentic relationships: The Five Love Languages, the Five Gates of Speech, and The Five-to-One Rule. (Hey, we thought the repetition of five things would help you put these into practice immediately.)

We recommend these practices to all our clients, as clear and loving communication creates trust and deeper connections. And for most of the women we know, when there is a strong foundation of trust with our sexual partners, we can open deeply and experience powerful and transcendent pleasure. In other words, yes, delicious orgasms—and also more peace and harmony in and out of the bedroom. And again, as you embody more of this pleasure, it will flow into all areas of your life. That is a wonderful gift to carry with you during your menopause.

The Five Love Languages is a best-selling, accessible book by Gary Chapman that explores how each of us prefers to experience and express our love. The five languages are:

1. Words of affirmation
2. Acts of service
3. Physical touch
4. Gift-giving
5. Quality time

Learning the love languages of yourself, your partner, and those closest to you—and offering love in a way that's deeply received—can bring profound happiness and ease into your life.

Julie

I love tuning into other people's love language. Pam's primary love language is acts of service. My favorite love language is gift-giving. But Pam doesn't care so much about gifts, so when I give her a gift, she appreciates it, but I'm not seeing and acknowledging her deepest need and what makes her feel loved. So the best way I can express my love for her is by showing up. I also listen or ask for what she needs to feel supported. Does she need help walking the dog while she makes a phone call? Can I stop by the grocery store for her and drop off ripe avocados? Acts of service. Not my thing, but hers. And she knows I love it when she gives me little presents. Identifying the love language of our dear ones and offering our love in a way that they can receive it makes our world a more loving and gentler place!

I also choose to practice, as much as possible, the Five Gates of Speech, which originate from Buddhist teachings. It is a mindful practice to choose your words wisely and to express yourself with loving kindness. The five gates are:

1. Is it true?
2. Is it kind?
3. Is it necessary?
4. Is it the right time?
5. Is it the right place?

You might be thinking, "Wow, then maybe I wouldn't be speaking much at all if I used these five gates as a filter." Yup, true, and probably not. We believe words have the power to create our reality. Choosing to speak with more self-awareness and intention does *not* mean you are a doormat. We feel more powerful and clear when we know that our words are truthful and have an impact. You may want to experiment with all of your relationships, *including* the way you speak to yourself. Most of us could also benefit from being more active and attentive listeners. Speaking less allows us to listen more.

Dr. John Gottman discovered from researching relationships that the difference between happy and unhappy couples is the balance between positive and negative interactions. Gottman found a very specific "magic ratio" of five to one, which means that for every negative interaction, a stable and happy relationship has five or more positive interactions. Negative interactions include being distant, emotionally dismissive, defensive, critical, or worse—attacking. Positive interactions include:

- Be interested
- Express affection
- Demonstrate they matter
- Intentional appreciation
- Find opportunities for agreement
- Empathize and apologize
- Accept your partner's perspective
- Laugh together

A fabulous taxi driver drove me to O'Hare Airport a couple of years ago. He shared that he had been married for more than forty years and that he still feels like he and his wife are newlyweds and remain very much in love. He said he treats her like a queen and compliments her every day. He shared that he had great respect for the work she does, how she mothered their children, and that their relationship was the most precious thing in his life. Well, I am certain they had the five love languages, five gates, and five-to-one ratio full-on in their marriage!

There are two wonderful experts we follow who offer deep insight and wisdom about intimate relationships. Esther Perel, psychotherapist and *New York Times* best-selling author of *Mating in Captivity: Unlocking Erotic Intelligence*, is recognized as one of today's most insightful and original voices on modern relationships. Terry Real is an internationally recognized family therapist, speaker, and *New York Times* best-seller of *Us: Getting Past You and Me to Build a More Loving Relationship*. Their books, online content, and teachings can support you in having a deeper understanding of creating and maintaining healthier love relationships.

Dating

"I am choosing, not waiting to be chosen."
—Jennifer Worman, Instagram@redsolesandredwine

Welcome to the exciting world of dating as a midlife woman! We are all about empowering you to embrace this new phase with confidence, self-assurance, and a sense of adventure. We have suggestions, tools, and some great stories to help you navigate midlife dating, and this includes dates with your current partner!

If you are single and ready to date, this may not sound sexy, but introspection is one of the keys to helping you find "your person." Midlife is such a great time to reignite old passions, rediscover what interests you, and nurture a healthy self-image. True confidence comes from knowing yourself and what makes you *you*. It's time to embrace the wisdom and experience you have acquired.

Why Midlife Is a Magical Chapter for Dating

Midlife can be the perfect time for finding love—or as I like to say, the perfect time to find "the lid to your pot!" With over 35 million singles over 50 in the U.S., the dating pool is deeper than many think! At this stage of life, we've weathered storms, grown through loss, and gained clarity about who we are—and what we truly want. The distractions of early adulthood—raising kids, building careers, chasing expectations—start to quiet down, making space for joy, fun, and meaningful connection.

This season is about intentional *choice*—where we live, how we love, and what happiness looks like. Whether you're interested in a deep, lasting partnership or a lighter, joyful companionship, the most important thing is to remember: you are the prize. The right person will make you feel safe, seen, and cherished—never confused or second-guessing. The love you find at midlife can be the best, most soul-filing love you will ever have! Become "psychotically optimistic" about your dating life—tell yourself that 'love will come to me, it's a when not an if!"

GETTING BACK OUT THERE AFTER A BREAKUP, DIVORCE, OR LOSS

Reentering the dating world after a long relationship can feel like jumping into the Atlantic ocean at midnight with no life vest on—but it can also be exhilarating. The key is intention. Just like you'd train for a marathon or plan a big trip, dating deserves a strategy.

Build a "dating trifecta":

1. Go digital: choose 1-2 quality dating apps and get familiar with the lay of the land.

2. Be visible IRL: go to events, try new hobbies, and engage with

people around you. Smile, offer a compliment, and watch people gravitate straight to you!

3. Tap your network: tell friends and colleagues you're open to being set up.

To make it even more fun, create a "Dating Board of Directors"—handpick 3-5 friends who are natural connectors and give them the VIP role of helping you meet someone wonderful. Make it playful, light, and full of possibilities. And when you're out and about, ditch the phone and radiate presence. Smile. Spark conversations. Magic often begins with a simple hello.

MAKING ONLINE DATING WORK FOR YOU

Online dating can feel like a jungle—or a goldmine—depending on your approach. When done well, it's one of the best ways to meet someone who matches your values and lifestyle. Start by choosing one or two apps that align with your goals. If one doesn't feel like a fit after a couple of months, switch it up. Dating is about momentum—not perfection.

Your photos are your first impression. Invest in bright, joyful images—especially a smiling headshot and full-body photo (ideally, you'll have six great photos to fit into the slots offered by most dating apps). Skip group pics and filters; people want to see you. Better yet, consider a lifestyle photo shoot that captures your personality in action—laughing at a café, strolling through a garden, or playing with your pup. Make sure you're looking right at the camera with a big smile on your face—people gravitate towards happy, warm people, and it's important that your photos show that! Avoid sunglasses which cover your eyes—the windows to your soul! And, look great in all of your photos—they should be well-lit and no more than one year old!

As for your bio? Don't write a novel—and most apps won't even allow that anymore. Many offer you around 200 characters which is less than two tweets! Use very short storytelling instead of self-promotion. Rather than saying, "I'm generous," try "I'll show up with homemade soup and your favorite movie when you're under the weather." Specific, sweet, and memorable. That's what stands out.

—BELA GANDHI,
Smart Dating Academy founder and president

We think there are some principles to consider regarding dating, and we love the book by Ali Binazir, the *Tao of Dating*.[174] It is a deep and satisfying dive into not just dating but intention setting and examining beliefs. It was recommended to us by a dear friend who is in a super amazing love relationship after a challenging marriage and an intense divorce. Below are some of Binazir's principles, with our own twist:

- **Have an abundance mindset,** seeing the world as full of possibility and an unlimited supply of goodness all around you. Binazir shares that even if only one-thousandth of 1% of the eight billion people in the world would be a fabulous match for you, that's 80,000 people. We mean, really... that's quite a dating pool!

- **Take good care of yourself.** Make yourself the priority. Our millennial friend Tinx, author of *The Shift* says, "The second you go on a crusade to change someone, you are elevating their importance in your life higher than your own. Nobody loves a fuckboi more than a big ol' ego that whispers in your ear, 'You could be the one to change him.'"[175] Short-term thinking usually leads to pain.

- **Be-do-have:** If you're a happy, loving, and generous person who takes good care of your body, mind, and spirit, doing activities you enjoy, then wonderful people will be attracted to you who enjoy being with you. Many people believe when you have the perfect partner, *then* you'll be happy. That's not how it works.

- **Feminine and masculine balance:** Feminine energy is yin—receptive, gentle, intuitive, and fulfilling. Yang is masculine energy—active, fast, fierce, and focused. Each of us has these qualities within us. Observe the balance of these energies in your relationships. Many people who have more feminine energy usually desire a more masculine partner, and femininity is often more desirable to the masculine. Binazir says, "Without polarity, relationships fall flat."[176] We know many powerful women who are more receptive and surrendered in their love relationships and lovemaking, as well as women who are the primary providers for their families and have chosen wonderful men who have more feminine energy and adore their women. There is something to this, so start observing your behavior out in the wild!

- **Take the time to know yourself.** This means perhaps learning to meditate, breathing, and connecting with yourself so that your ego or false self doesn't rule your life and lead you into unhappy situations. Open up and make space for love. Love always wins.

Before we talk about finding your person, we encourage you to grab a journal and take some time to reflect on your past relationships. Consider what has worked and what hasn't. Did you learn any lessons from your past relationships? Did the gifts of these lessons give you a deeper understanding of yourself and what you are looking for? Taking the time to consider your answers to these questions will help you to more clearly define what you *do* want.

One of the most powerful things you can do is create your list. What do we mean by this? Earlier in this chapter, we talked about the reticular activating system. Can this work for dating, too? Well, hell yes! You are more likely to attract what you want if you know what you want. Many women have told us what they don't want. Make your list of what you *do* want. Get super clear. Envision your perfect person. What do they look like? What qualities do they have that you admire? What do you see yourself doing with this person? Get into the description and write it down. Envision your future self. What interests are you sharing? Imagine your day-to-day life with this person. They are having conversations with you, sleeping next to you, and yes, you can even imagine your love making! Feel it all. Experience it all. See it all.

If you want a really powerful exercise, you can "future pull" your person. By future pulling, we mean pulling your future toward you! Oh yes—it works! You can talk, write, and act as if your person is already in your presence. For example, on your list, say, "I love that my person is always making me laugh. I love that my person is kind and generous. I love that we do amazing things together and that we are always having adventures. I am the best version of myself with my person." You get the picture—literally! And extra points for getting into the details.

If you're game, let's talk manifesting mastery—you came here to upgrade, right? When you envision your future love, ask yourself, "Am I a match with my person?" Let's be real here: You may have some personal work to do to manifest the right partner. "Have I developed myself in a way that will attract my ideal person?" This can look like releasing old patterns and beliefs and becoming the best version of yourself. We are going to encourage you to dive deep.

> At fifty, our client Trish finally left her loveless marriage. Even though it was painful for her, she remained in the marriage for the children. And for years, she said every day, "I want to know what being in love feels like." She knew her husband was not in love with her, and she was not in love with him. Trish longed for respect, admiration, and appreciation, which wasn't present in her marriage. She became very clear about what she desired in a future relationship. Not long after her divorce was finalized, her college boyfriend reached out because of her status update on Facebook (haha). They met at a restaurant, and when she saw him, she knew all bets were off. It was as if no time had passed, and she instantly knew he was the one. Trish had thought of him for years, as he had also thought of her. Within a year, they were married, and they both feel very fortunate to have found the love of their lives.

Trish and her current husband have discussed and wondered if they could have made it as a couple in college. They both agree that they had to go through difficult relationships so they could appreciate and value the amazing relationship they have now. Ten years later, they are still deeply in love and blissfully married. Interestingly enough, in her book *Late Love: Mating in Maturity*, Avivah Wittenberg-Cox wrote, "Many people who leave a spouse end up with a friend. There is an immediate sense of trust and shared history."[177]

Be open to being surprised! The person you are looking for could be someone you already know. Maybe it's an old love, a childhood friend, a former colleague, your high school prom date, or even someone from your gym. We have heard it all, and you just never know.

As midlife women, we can learn something from the younger generation. And let's face it, a lot of us have no experience with digital dating, texting/sexting, or how to even create an online dating profile. Tinx, the millennial author, shares that you should take your focus off the other person and bring your attention back to yourself. What are *you* looking for? What do *you* want? Don't fall in love with potential. Albert Einstein reportedly said, "Women marry men hoping they will change, and men marry women hoping they will not." So each is inevitably disappointed. And often, the big change for us is in midlife!

You have the power to go out there and make things happen. So, my dears, make your list. Then put it away. Yup—put it away and know that you have put your order in. Then go do what brings you joy and lights you up. You will naturally radiate more confidence and more of your juiciness. If you want to get things moving along, it will help to take an action step. Taking an action step will deliver a message: You're ready.

Pam was in sales for many years, and her theory on dating is that it's a numbers game. In sales, you make so many cold calls to get a few leads, to get a couple of appointments until you finally get your sale! Along the way, you get more comfortable, improve your sales skills, and eventually make your numbers. Wink, wink. So make your "cold calls." You may want to start by getting some girlfriends together and creating your online dating profile. If you find someone you like, make a date "appointment" and get a dating pool going. Continue to date other people. Especially if you haven't dated in this century (haha), you have to get comfortable with dating and meeting new people. Keep practicing.

> Janie had been divorced for six years and finally decided she wanted to start dating. She was set up on five blind dates by five different friends, and unfortunately, none of them went well. Because of her age, Janie was very reluctant to try online dating. She was seriously concerned about the exposure and meeting people that she knew nothing about. But at the age of fifty-eight, she mustered up her courage because she wanted to meet a wonderful partner, and finally went for it. She had her besties take pictures of her doing things she loved—gardening, tending to her flowers, and playing paddle ball—and they helped her build an online profile.
>
> She went on a bunch of dates, but after every date, she was ghosted. What was up? She was stuck in a pattern of picking the wrong guys. And you know what was missing? *The list.* She met with a good friend who encouraged her to deeply review the qualities she was looking for in a partner and then make her list. When she and her friend were reviewing her list together, her friend asked if her former husband had any of those qualities. He had none. That realization is what finally broke her pattern of attracting the wrong people. On the very next date, she met her new husband. He was wonderful, attentive, loving, and loved the same activities she did. It's been several years now, and Janie says she couldn't be happier now that she has found her beloved match.

No matter how guarded you may have become after a failed relationship, a lost friendship, or a waning marriage, know that you always have the power and wisdom to create your future. Good things don't always come when or as we expect them to; however, if you take time to nurture self-love, tend to the old wounds, and be open and welcoming to new connections, something special awaits you. Trust yourself, love openly, and expect the unexpected.

CONCLUSION

What have you learned here? A lot, we hope.

We wrote this book to empower *you*. It's like Glinda told Dorothy in *The Wizard of Oz*, "You've always had the power, my dear. You just had to learn it for yourself." You have the ruby slippers. Now is the time to claim your power and choose to live your life with confidence and joy.

We wrote this book for you because, as you have learned from all of our stories, we struggled to find the answers for ourselves. We wanted to share what has helped us in the hopes that it might help you too. And if you are still in the trenches, we hope the wisdom in this book gives you the confidence to take action and know the answers are out there. You don't have to suffer needlessly. You have every right to live a healthy and beautiful life.

We also wrote this book because we are still living in a patriarchal world where women's health concerns are readily dismissed, and there is still an enormous amount of work to do. We are outraged by the lack of research regarding the aging female body. We are frustrated that the word "menopause" is still whispered as if it's shameful. We celebrate every woman who is bringing the truth into the open—their stories, their wisdom, and their research. They inspire us! You know, it takes a lot of courage to live in a female body.

"Menopause gets a really bad rap and needs some rebranding."
—Gwenyth Paltrow

"What a woman's body is taking her through is important information. It's an important thing to take up space in a society because half of us are going through this, but we're living like it's not happening."
—Michelle Obama

"*Perimenopause and menopause should be treated as the rites of passage they are . . . if not celebrated, then at least accepted and acknowledged and honored.*"
—Gillian Anderson

"*Embrace the changes taking place. They will take you and your life to someplace new, someplace you can't fully imagine now because it's so different from where you have been.*"
—Melody Beattie

The midlife and menopause discussion is evolving every day, week, month, and to be fair, we don't have all the answers. Yet. By reading this book and sharing it with others, you are elevating the conversation, which is so desperately needed. Keep the faith though—we are definitely moving forward. We must ensure that future generations of women have a gentler, more supportive, and safer midlife experience than previous ones.

Once you get your s**t together, and you will, how can you lift others? The bottom line is that we have to join hands and take care of one another. By fostering a collective strength, all women are uplifted. Solidarity among women is a force that can break barriers and reshape narratives. Goodness knows we need that.

Remember, we did the research before writing this book. The topics covered were the topics women wanted to know more about. Now that you know that, start having conversations with your friends about what's going on with you. Odds are they too are looking for someone to share with and to see them where they are. Women deserve to be accepted and celebrated at all times in our lives.

Ladies, no lifeboats are coming to rescue us. It's up to us to demand better care from our providers, support more funding for research, get insurance companies to cover *all* perimenopausal and menopausal care, take better care of our bodies, and support other women in every way that we can.

A midlife upgrade is not for the weak of heart. Staying open and trusting the journey can be challenging when the path is uncharted and unclear. Yet opportunities abound if you're willing to have faith that there's purpose in the process. You're going someplace new!

Our chaotic world aches for the return of the divine feminine. We've spent thousands of years under a paradigm that has failed to honor women —and now, more than ever, the wisdom of the midlife woman is needed. It's time for all of us to rise and claim our power.

Let's rebrand this stage of life and imagine what's possible. Because you are not done—not even close.

You are loved.

You are valued.

You are needed.

You are *upgraded*.

Scan this code to access our exclusive BOOK PORTAL packed with powerful resources, inspiring playlists, guided meditations, and more. And don't stop there—you're also invited to join our Midlife Upgrade community and course, where real transformation and connection begins!

ACKNOWLEDGMENTS

Thank you to all of our many clients and friends who have generously and courageously shared their midlife journeys. You have been the inspiration for this book and helped bring it to life.

We are eternally grateful to all scientists, physicians, health practitioners, healers, coaches, and every human who is dedicated to uplifting the lives of women.

To those unpacking midlife and menopause, who've added their wisdom and experience to the conversation, thank you for your contributions. Your work is not only shattering taboos but is paving the way for a brighter, more informed, and inclusive future for all women.

Our gratitude to our brilliant physician friends and supporters, Shanhong Lu, MD, PhD; Vesna Skul, MD, FACP; Danuta Hoyer, MD; and Rose Kumar, MD. Each of you has always been ahead of the curve advocating for women, speaking truth to power, and treating your patients with great compassion and impeccable care.

Thank you to the wonderful women that contributed to this book—Amy Owen, Barri Leiner Grant, Donna Kendrick and Bela Gandhi.

A big thank you with all of our hearts to some of the wonderful and brilliant women dedicated to cracking the code on menopause and midlife! Lucky for us, many have become dear friends: Kelly Casperson, MD; Cindy Eckert; Tamsen Fadal; Heidi Flagg, MD; Shieva Ghofrany, MD; Suzanne Gilberg, MD; Rebbecca Hertel, DO; Somi Javaid, MD; Christine Kress, DNP; Sharon Malone, MD; Corinne Menn, MD; Aoife O'Sullivan, MD; Jackie Piasta, NP; Heather Quaile, DNP; Sameena Rahman, MD; Jila Senemar, MD; Kate White, MD.

Thank you to our wonderful BFFs, Jennifer and Penny, who graciously agreed to be beta readers.

Thank you to Sara Connell, Founder of Thought Leader Academy. From the first moment we heard you speak in October 2022; you blew our minds and hearts wide open. You held our hands, saw what we couldn't see, and encouraged us when our inner gremlins tried to take us out. You are the real deal. This book was created because of your faith in us.

Thank you to Marsha Craig, who told us we had to meet Sara and gifted us an invitation to a Thought Leader event. Without you dear Marsha, there would be no book.

To our magical senior editor, Audrey Fierberg, who went above and beyond to bring this book to life. And also to editors Hannah Rumsey and Mary Nelligan, thank you for coaching a couple of newbies.

A deep gratitude to our lovely and talented illustrator, Clara Baumgarten. Her illustrations truly honored the beauty of the female anatomy.

Thank you to Claudine Mansour for saving the day at the final hour and helping us create the book of our dreams.

To the amazing women in our Thought Leader Academy Mastery pod. You are an inspiration for all women. Thank you for believing in us!

Pamela

To my dearest daughter, Hannah. Since the minute you were born, I knew you would be my greatest teacher, and that has held true. I'm so lucky you chose me as your mom. I want your journey to be easier than mine.

To my loving husband, Jim. You always have my back, and your love, support, and encouragement have meant the world to me.

To my daughters in love, Morgan and Francesca, for your acceptance and love. I won the step-parent lottery with you two.

To my mother, for being the strong woman you are and for always believing in me.

To Jennifer, who knew my love of all things health and food and talked me into being a health coach.

I have been lucky to have an amazing tribe of women in my life who have been my confidants, guides and biggest cheerleaders. Many of you have held space for me and wiped my tears in my darkest moments. I cannot even begin to tell you how grateful I am for your years of love and support. Allison, Nicole, Danusia, Vesna, Ellen, Lindsey, Kristi, Kelly, Michelle, Christy, Joanne, Angela, Liz, and Jackie . . . just to name a few.

Julie

My deepest gratitude to all of the invincible women in my life, many of whom I met when I was entering midlife. A circle of women is an essential survival tool for the menopausal journey, and each of you has loved me up, dusted me off, and helped me stand tall in my strength and power. Thank you for your prayers, faith, dinners, wild adventures, and for holding me in my grief, as well as my happiness. I love each of you so very much. I would not be here without you.

To my LiFT goddesses, TLA inspiring women, Mama Gena sisters, Montessori moms, and meditation friends.

To my ride or die crew, Alison, Andrea, Annicka, Barb, Donna, JulieAnn, Kate, Kathy, Linda, Michelle, Penny, Preeti, Rachel, Renee, Sara, Stephanie, Shanhong, and Wini. Sh*t, we've been through a lot together! Thank you for being my soul family. Let the good times roll. We deserve it!

To my brilliant grandmother, Baba, my elegant, trailblazing mother, Margaret, my beloved Aunt Charlene, who always had my back, and my powerhouse sister, Sara. You are my family. I will always love you.

And to the enlightened men who have been cheering me on. . .

My dearest son, Ram. Thank you for choosing me as your mother. You are the greatest blessing of my life. Continue to shine your light. I am so very grateful that you have the utmost reverence and appreciation for strong women—and all women. You are leading the way for your generation of men. I love you more. P.S. Thank you for creating the beautiful book cover for us!

And to my "wasbund," Daniel, for your infinite love and for sharing your grace and wisdom with me for thirty years. Thank you for always seeing me as beautiful. It was a good run. Loving you.

NOTES

CHAPTER 1

1 Thayer, Colette, and Cheryl Lampkin. "Perimenopause Is More Than Hot Flashes: What Women Need to Know." AARP, 4 May 2021, www.aarp.org/pri/topics/health/conditions-treatment/perimenopause-hormonal-changes-impact.html.

2 Cleveland Clinic. "Perimenopause: Symptoms, Causes, Diagnosis, Treatment, and Prevention." *Cleveland Clinic*, https://my.clevelandclinic.org/health/diseases/21608-perimenopause. Accessed 18 Apr. 2025.

3 World Health Organization. "Menopause." World Health Organization, 16 Oct. 2024, https://www.who.int/news-room/fact-sheets/detail/menopause.

4 Bonafide. 2021. State of Menopause Survey. Accessed May 8, 2024. https://hellobonafide.com/pages/state-of-menopause.

5 Ebert, Morgan. "Study: Perimenopause Symptoms Common in Women as Young as 30." Contemporary OB/GYN, 27 Feb. 2025, www.contemporaryobgyn.net/view/study-perimenopause-symptoms-common-in-women-as-young-as-30.

6 Kindra. "Menopause Medical Misdiagnosis: One in Three Women Misdiagnosed with Menopause Symptoms." *Kindra*, 6 Oct. 2023, https://ourkindra.com/blogs/journal/menopause-medical-misdiagnosis?srsltid=AfmBOor1l-3SABRTAGZuI3MpryjTsx-vHvDv46QH1Su-0YvO51D4wInJi.

7 Women's Health in Focus at NIH. 2022. "Research on Menopause ." National Institutes of Health. July. Accessed May 6, 2024. https://orwh.od.nih.gov/sites/orwh/files/docs/ORWHInFocus52_508.pdf.

8 Hopkins Medicine. "Study: Fewer Than One in Five Doctors Receive Menopause Training." The Johns Hopkins Gazette, 5 June 2013, https://hub.jhu.edu/gazette/2013/june/news-menopause-medicine-training-needed/.

9   Johns Hopkins Medicine. 2024. Introduction to Menopause. Accessed May 8, 2024. https://www.hopkinsmedicine.org/health/conditions-and-diseases/introduction-to-menopause#:~:text=Hot%20flashes%20or%20flushes%20are,for%202%20years%20or%20less

10 Venborg, Emilie, et al. "The Association Between Postpartum Depression and Perimenopausal Depression: A Nationwide Register-Based Cohort Study." Maturitas, vol. 169, 2023, pp. 10–15. https://doi.org/10.1016/j.maturitas.2022.12.001.

11 Fadal, T. (2025). *How to Menopause: Take Charge of Your Health, Reclaim Your Life, and Feel Even Better than Before.* Hachette Go.

12 Kapoor, Ekta. "Weight Gain in Women at Midlife: A Concise Review of the Pathophysiology and Strategies for Management." Mayo Clinic Proceedings, vol. 92, no. 10, 2017, pp. 1552-1558. https://doi.org/10.1016/j.mayocp.2017.07.011.

13 "Brain Fog." Let's Talk Menopause, 2025, www.letstalkmenopause.org/our-articles/brain-fog.

CHAPTER 2

14 Wang, Y., Li, Y., & Zhang, X. (2021). Factors affecting the risk of postpartum hemorrhage in pregnant women. *BMC Pregnancy and Childbirth*, 21, Article 123. https://doi.org/10.1186/s12884-021-03678-9

15 Belluck, Pam. 2023. "FDA Approves First Pill for Postpartum Depression." The New York Times. August 4. Accessed May 7, 2024. https://www.nytimes.com/2023/08/04/health/postpartum-depression-pill-fda.html.

16 "Postpartum disorder." *Wikipedia*, 10 June 2024, https://en.wikipedia.org/wiki/Postpartum_disorder. Accessed 10 June 2024.

17 Pert, Candace B. *Molecules of Emotion: The Science Behind Mind-Body Medicine.* New York: Scribner, 1997.

18 Dalton, Katharina; Holton, Wendy. *Depression After Childbirth: How to Recognize, Treat, and Prevent Postnatal Depression.* Oxford University Press. 2001

19 Gross, Rachel E.. *Vagina Obscura: An Anatomical Voyage.* W.W. Norton & Co. 2022

20 Romm, A. (n.d.). *Overlooked & Ignored: Why Women Don't Get a Thyroid Diagnosis.* Retrieved from https://avivaromm.com/

hypothyroidism-feminist-issue/::contentReference{index=2}

21   Romm, A. (n.d.). *Overlooked & Ignored: Why Women Don't Get a Thyroid Diagnosis*. Retrieved from https://avivaromm.com/hypothyroidism-feminist-issue/::contentReference{index=2}

22   Liu, Yun-Zi, Yun-Xia Wang, and Chun-Lei Jiang. "Inflammation: The Common Pathway of Stress-Related Diseases." Frontiers in Human Neuroscience, vol. 11, 2017, p. 316.

23   Findlay, J. K., Hutt, K. J., Hickey, M., & Anderson, R. A. (2022). How is the number of oocytes in the human ovary regulated? *Cell and Tissue Research*, 387(3), 505–519. https://doi.org/10.1007/s00441-021-03560-5

24   American College of Obstetricians and Gynecologists. (2014). *Female age-related fertility decline* (Committee Opinion No. 589). https://www.acog.org/clinical/clinical-guidance/committee-opinion/articles/2014/03/female-age-related-fertility-decline

25   "United States—Life Expectancy at Birth, Female (Years)." Trading Economics, 2025, https://tradingeconomics.com/united-states/life-expectancy-at-birth-female-years-wb-data.html.

26   Greenwood, V. (2023, October 19). *The secrets of aging are hidden in your ovaries*. Wired. Retrieved April 23, 2025, from https://www.wired.com/story/aging-menopause-longevity/

27   Robbins, Tony, Peter H. Diamandis, and Robert Hariri. Life Force: How New Breakthroughs in Precision Medicine Can Transform the Quality of Your Life & Those You Love. Simon & Schuster, 2022.

28   Ghanemi, A., Yoshioka, M., & St-Amand, J. (2022). Exercise, diet and sleeping as regenerative medicine adjuvants: Obesity and ageing as illustrations. *Medicines*, 9(1), 7. https://doi.org/10.3390/medicines9010007::contentReference{index=1}

29   Gjerstad, J. K., Lightman, S. L., and Spiga, F. "Role of Glucocorticoid Negative Feedback in the Regulation of HPA Axis Pulsatility." *Stress*, vol. 21, no. 5, 2018, pp. 403–416. https://doi.org/10.1080/10253890.2018.1470238::contentReference{index=2}

30   "Returning to Work." 4th Trimester Project, NewMomHealth.com, 2025, newmomhealth.com/selfcare/returning-to-work/#:~:text=One%20out%20of%20every%20four,or%20full%2Dtime%20employment%20smoother.

31 World Health Organization. (2019). *Trends in maternal mortality: 2000 to 2017*. https://www.who.int/reproductivehealth/publications/maternal-mortality-2000-2017/en/

32 U.S. Food and Drug Administration. (2019, March 19). *FDA approves first treatment for post-partum depression*. Retrieved from https://www.fda.gov/news-events/press-announcements/fda-approves-first-treatment-post-partum-depression

33 Dalton, Katharina. Depression After Childbirth: How to Recognize and Treat Postnatal Illness. 2nd ed., Oxford University Press, 1989.

CHAPTER 3

34 Rutherford, Erin. "The Change of Life: Menopause and Our Changing Perspectives." The Devil's Tale, 23 Mar. 2018, blogs.library.duke.edu/rubenstein/2018/03/23/the-change-of-life-menopause-and-our-changing-perspectives/.

35 International Menopause Society. (2024). *Menopause and MHT in 2024: Addressing the key controversies—an International Menopause Society White Paper*. https://www.imsociety.org/wp-content/uploads/2024/09/Menopause-and-MHT-in-2024-addressing-the-key-controversies-an-International-Menopause-Society-White-Paper.pdf

36 Mayo Clinic Health System. (2021, November 30). *Pausing to learn more about menopause*. https://www.mayoclinichealthsystem.org/hometown-health/speaking-of-health/too-embarrassed-to-ask-part-3

37 Shen, W. (2018). Nearly one-third of this country's women are postmenopausal, and many of them are needlessly suffering. In *AARP Recognizes Menopause Care Gap*. HealthyWomen. Retrieved from https://www.healthywomen.org/your-health/menopause-aging-well/aarp-recognizes-menopause-care-gap::contentReference{index=4}

38 AARP. (2018). *Menopause experiences: Providers can do better in educating women*. https://www.aarp.org/pri/topics/health/conditions-treatment/menopause-experiences-healthcare/

39 Malone, S. (2024). *Grown woman talk: Your guide to getting and staying healthy*. Crown Publishing Group.

40 Malone, S. (2024). *Grown woman talk: Your guide to getting and staying healthy*. Crown Publishing Group.

41 Johns Hopkins Medicine. (n.d.). *Estrogen's Effects on the Female Body*. Retrieved April 22, 2025, from https://www.hopkinsmedicine.org/health/conditions-and-diseases/estrogens-effects-on-the-female-body

42 Haver, Mary Claire MD. 2024. The New Menopause. Rodale Publisher. PG 4

43 Iverson, Ben. "Middle-Aged Men Can Blame Estrogen, Too." The New York Times, 11 Sept. 2013, www.nytimes.com/2013/09/12/science/middle-aged-men-can-blame-estrogen-too.html.

44 National Heart, Lung, and Blood Institute. "Women's Health Initiative (WHI)." National Institutes of Health, U.S. Department of Health & Human Services, 2025, www.nhlbi.nih.gov/science/womens-health-initiative-whi.

45 UCLA Health. (2022, June 15). *2002 HRT study comes under criticism*. https://www.uclahealth.org/news/article/2002-hrt-study-comes-under-criticism

46 National Heart, Lung, and Blood Institute. (n.d.). *Women's Health Initiative (WHI)*. https://www.nhlbi.nih.gov/science/womens-health-initiative-whi

47 NPR. (2013, October 4). *The last word on hormone therapy from the Women's Health Initiative*. https://www.npr.org/sections/health-shots/2013/10/04/229171477/the-last-word-on-hormone-therapy-from-the-womens-health-initiative

48 Women's Health Concern. (2022, November). *HRT: Benefits and risks* [PDF]. https://www.womens-health-concern.org/wp-content/uploads/2022/12/11-WHC-FACTSHEET-HRT-BenefitsRisks-NOV2022-B.pdf

49 Langer, R. D. (2017). The evidence base for HRT: what can we believe? *Climacteric*, 20(2), 91–96. https://doi.org/10.1080/13697137.2017.1280251

50 Casperson, Kelly. *You Are Not Broken: Stop "Should-ing" All Over Your Sex Life*. YANB MEDIA, 2022.

51 Ribeiro, Luísa Silva de Carvalho, et al. "Breaking Bad News in Obstetrics and Gynecology: We Must Talk About It." Revista Brasileira de Ginecologia e Obstetrícia, vol. 44, no. 6, 2022, pp. 621–628. https://doi.org/10.1055/s-0042-1742316.

52 Dominus, Susan. "Women Have Been Misled About Menopause." The New York Times Magazine, 1 Feb. 2023, www.nytimes.com/2023/02/01/magazine/menopause-hot-flashes-hormone-therapy.html.

53 American College of Obstetricians and Gynecologists. "Management of Menopausal Symptoms." Practice Bulletin No. 141, Jan. 2014, www.acog.org/clinical/clinical-guidance/practice-bulletin/articles/2014/01/management-of-menopausal-symptoms.

54 Attia, Peter. 2022. "Menstruation, Menopause, and Hormone Replacement Therapy for Women." YouTube, August 20.

55 Gilberg-Lenz, Suzanne. "Don't Fear the Hot Flash: Menopause Isn't a Disease —But It Is a Health Issue We Need to Talk About." Salon, 13 Nov. 2022, www.salon.com/2022/11/13/dont-fear-the-hot-flash-menopause-isnt-a-disease-but-it-is-a-health-issue-we-need-to-talk-about/.

56 Bone Health & Osteoporosis Foundation. (n.d.). *What women need to know.* https://www.bonehealthandosteoporosis.org/preventing-fractures/general-facts/what-women-need-to-know/

57 Dam, T. V., Dalgaard, L. B., Ringgaard, S., Johansen, F. T., Bengtsen, M. B., Mose, M., Lauritsen, K. M., Ørtenblad, N., Gravholt, C. H., & Hansen, M. (2021). Transdermal estrogen therapy improves gains in skeletal muscle mass after 12 weeks of resistance training in early postmenopausal women. *Frontiers in Physiology, 11,* 596130. https://doi.org/10.3389/fphys.2020.596130

58 Hansen, M., Kongsgaard, M., Holm, L., Skovgaard, D., Magnusson, S. P., Qvortrup, K., Larsen, J. O., Aagaard, P., Dahl, M., Serup, A., Koskinen, S., Kjaer, M., & Langberg, H. (2009). Effect of estrogen on tendon collagen synthesis, tendon structural characteristics, and biomechanical properties in postmenopausal women. *Journal of Applied Physiology, 106*(4), 1385–1393. https://doi.org/10.1152/japplphysiol.90935.2008

59 Xie, F., & Li, X. (2022). Estrogen mediates an atherosclerotic-protective action via estrogen receptor alpha/SREBP-1 signaling. *Frontiers in Cardiovascular Medicine, 9,* 9294214. https://doi.org/10.3389/fcvm.2022.9294214

60 Cleveland Clinic. (n.d.). *Estrogen-Dependent Cancers: Causes, Diagnosis & Treatment.* Retrieved April 22, 2025, from https://my.clevelandclinic.org/health/diseases/10312-estrogen-dependent-cancers

61   Lazarou, J. (2013, June). Study: OB/GYNs need menopause medicine training. *Johns Hopkins University Gazette*. https://hub.jhu.edu/gazette/2013/june/news-menopause-medicine-training-needed/

62   Van Amburg, Jessie. "Nearly 1 in 3 Women Have Had Their Menopause Symptoms Misdiagnosed." Kindra Journal, 2023, ourkindra.com/blogs/journal/menopause-medical-misdiagnosis.

63   Casperson, Kelly. *You Are Not Broken: Stop "Should-ing" All Over Your Sex Life*. YANB MEDIA, 2022.

64   de Beauvoir, Simone. The Second Sex. Translated by Constance Borde and Sheila Malovany-Chevallier, Vintage Books, 2011.

CHAPTER 4

65   Stock, Wendy. "Women's Sexual Desire—Disordered or Misunderstood?" Sex Therapy Frameworks and Sexual Problems, Dysfunctions, and Disorders, Dec. 2021, ResearchGate, doi:10.13140/RG.2.2.36414.64327.

66   "Attraction Differences Between Men and Women." TwoPlusTwo Forums, 3 Apr. 2009, forumserver.twoplustwo.com/63/lounge-discussion-review/attraction-differences-between-men-women-451529/.

67   Thomashauer, Regena. *Pussy: A Reclamation*. Hay House LLC, 2018.

68   American Psychiatric Association. (1980). *Diagnostic and statistical manual of mental disorders* (3rd ed.). Washington, DC: Author.

69   Casperson, Kelly. *You Are Not Broken: Stop "Should-ing" All Over Your Sex Life*. YANB MEDIA, 2022.

70   Lindberg, Laura D., and Leslie M. Kantor. "Adolescents' Receipt of Sex Education in a Nationally Representative Sample, 2011–2019." Journal of Adolescent Health, vol. 70, no. 2, Feb. 2022, pp. 290–297. Elsevier, doi:10.1016/j.jadohealth.2021.08.027.

71   Thomashauer, Regena. *Pussy: A Reclamation*. Hay House LLC, 2018.

72   Ginsberg, R. L., Tinker, L., Liu, J., Gray, J., Sangi-Haghpeykar, H., Manson, J. E., & Rossouw, J. E. (2016). Prevalence and correlates of body image dissatisfaction in postmenopausal women. *Women & Health*, 56(1), 23–47. https://doi.org/10.1080/03630242.2015.1074636;:contentReference{index=1}

73   Dunn, Jancee. *Hot and Bothered: What No One Tells You About Menopause and How to Feel Like Yourself Again*. G.P Putnam's Sons. 2023

74 Foria Wellness. (n.d.). *Vulva mapping: A guide to female sexual anatomy*. Foria. Retrieved April 23, 2025, from https://www.foriawellness.com/blogs/learn/vulva-mapping-guide-to-female-sexual-anatomy

75 International Society for Sexual Medicine. (2020). *How long does it take a woman to reach orgasm?* Retrieved April 24, 2025, from https://www.issm.info/sexual-health-qa/how-long-does-it-take-a-woman-to-reach-orgasm

76 Brincat, Clarissa. 2022. "Why is the clit so sensitive? Thanks to over 10,000 nerves, first real count finds." Medical News Today. November 3. Accessed May 8, 2024. https://www.medicalnewstoday.com/articles/why-is-the-clit-so-sensitive-thanks-to-over-10000-nerves-first-real-count-finds.

77 O'Connell, H. E., Sanjeevan, K. V., & Hutson, J. M. (2005). Anatomy of the clitoris. *The Journal of Urology*, 174(4 Pt 1), 1189–1195.

78 Faught, B. (2023, August 15). *The benefits of having sex after menopause*. Bonafide Health. Retrieved April 23, 2025, from https://hellobonafide.com/blogs/news/the-benefits-of-having-sex-after-menopause

79 Wheeler, C. (2022, July 27). *Stop Faking It with Vella Bioscience* [Audio podcast episode]. In K. & K. (Hosts), *Fuck IT ALL™ feat. I AM Radio*. IT ALL Media. https://itallpodcast.buzzsprout.com/1410724/episodes/10987239-stop-faking-it-with-vella-bioscience

80 Morse, E. (2023, September 28). The secret to productivity is pleasure, according to this sex expert. *GQ*. Retrieved April 23, 2025, from https://www.gq.com/story/routine-excellence-emily-morse:contentReference{index=1}

81 Abramović, M. (2024, October 8). 'Women give me babies to hold. I'm loved!' Marina Abramović on art, ageing and being bigger than Trump. *The Guardian*. Retrieved April 23, 2025, from https://www.theguardian.com/artanddesign/2024/oct/08/women-give-me-babies-to-hold-im-loved-marina-abramovic-on-art-ageing-and-being-bigger-than-trump

82 Faught, B. (n.d.). *The Benefits of Having Sex After Menopause*. Bonafide Health. Retrieved from https://hellobonafide.com/blogs/news/the-benefits-of-having-sex-after-menopause

83 Health Europa. (2019, September 9). *Survey shows menopausal women being prescribed inappropriate antidepressants*. Health Europa. Retrieved April 23, 2025, from https://www.healtheuropa.com/survey-shows-menopausal-women-being-prescribed-inappropriate-antidepressants/94110/

84   Comella, Lynn. Vibrator Nation: How Feminist Sex-Toy Stores Changed the Business of Pleasure. Duke University Press, 2017.

85   "The Yoni Egg: A Key to Female Energy, Inner Beauty, and Self-Confidence." InnerSelf, 2021, innerself.com/personal/relationships/couples/sexuality/24673-the-yoni-egg-key-to-female-energy-inner-beauty-and-self-confidence.html.

86   Shifren, J. L., Monz, B. U., Russo, P. A., Segreti, A., & Johannes, C. B. (2008). Sexual problems and distress in United States women: Prevalence and correlates. *Obstetrics & Gynecology*, 112(5), 970–978. https://doi.org/10.1097/AOG.0b013e3181898cdb

87   The Menopause Society. (n.d.). *Pain with penetration*. https://www.menopause.org/for-women/sexual-health-menopause-online/sexual-problems-at-midlife/pain-with-penetration

88   Rahn, David D., et al. "Vaginal Estrogen for Genitourinary Syndrome of Menopause: A Systematic Review." Obstetrics & Gynecology, vol. 124, no. 6, 2014, pp. 1147–1156. PubMed Central, https://pmc.ncbi.nlm.nih.gov/articles/PMC4855283/.

89   Let's Talk Menopause. (n.d.). *Symptom Spotlight: Painful Sex*. Retrieved April 23, 2025, from https://www.letstalkmenopause.org/our-articles/symptom-spotlight-painful-sex

90   Raz, R., & Stamm, W. E. (1993). A controlled trial of intravaginal estriol in postmenopausal women with recurrent urinary tract infections. *New England Journal of Medicine*, 329(11), 753–756. https://doi.org/10.1056/NEJM199309093291102

91   Casperson, K. (2024, March 11). *Dr. Kelly's Guide to Affordable Vaginal Hormone Therapy*. Retrieved April 21, 2025, from https://kellycaspersonmd.com/dr-kellys-guide-to-affordable-hormone-therapy/::contentReference{index=1}

92   Womaness. 2022. Ask A Doctor: "Why Does Sex Hurt Now?" It's more common than you think. Dr. Somi Javaid of HerMD tells you why. October 26. Accessed May 8, 2024. https://womaness.com/blogs/blog/ask-a-doctor-why-does-sex-hurt-now.

93   Urbaniak, Kasia. *Unbound: A Woman's Guide to Power*. TarcherPerigee. 2021.

94   Casperson, Kelly. *You Are Not Broken: Stop "Should-ing" All Over Your Sex Life*. YANB MEDIA, 2022.

CHAPTER 5

95 Mayo Clinic Staff. "Sleep Tips: 6 Steps to Better Sleep." Mayo Clinic, 7 May 2022, www.mayoclinic.org/healthy-lifestyle/adult-health/in-depth/sleep/art-20048379.

96 Neilson, Susie. 2019. "A Warm Bedtime Bath Can Help You Cool Down And Sleep Better." NPR. July 25. Accessed May 7, 2024. https://www.npr.org/sections/health-shots/2019/07/25/745010965/a-warm-bedtime-bath-can-help-you-cool-down-and-sleep-better.

97 Hendler, R. A., Ramchandani, V. A., Gilman, J., & Hommer, D. W. (2013). Stimulant and sedative effects of alcohol. Current topics in behavioral neurosciences, 13, 489–509. https://doi.org/10.1007/7854_2011_135

98 Sleep Foundation. (n.d.). *Why Do We Need Sleep?* Retrieved April 21, 2025, from https://www.sleepfoundation.org/how-sleep-works/why-do-we-need-sleep::contentReference{index=2}

99 Centers for Disease Control and Prevention. (2016, February 18). *1 in 3 adults don't get enough sleep*. https://archive.cdc.gov/www_cdc_gov/media/releases/2016/p0215-enough-sleep.html

100 Baker, F. C., Willoughby, A. R., Sassoon, S. A., Colrain, I. M., & de Zambotti, M. (2015). Insomnia in women approaching menopause: Beyond perception. *Menopause*, 22(7), 708–716. https://doi.org/10.1097/GME.0000000000000365

101 Taavoni, S., Ekbatani, N., Kashaniyan, M., & Haghani, H. (2011). Effect of valerian on sleep quality in postmenopausal women: a randomized placebo-controlled clinical trial. Menopause (New York, N.Y.), 18(9), 951–955. https://doi.org/10.1097/gme.0b013e31820e9acf

102 Gibson, C. J., et al. (2020, September 28). *Cannabis use for menopause symptom management among midlife women veterans*. Presented at the 2020 Virtual Annual Meeting of The North American Menopause Society. Retrieved from https://www.contemporaryobgyn.net/view/cannabis-for-managing-menopause-symptoms

103 Berman, Michelle. "Cannabis May Offer Relief from Menopause Symptoms: What to Know." Verywell Health, 25 Oct. 2022, www.verywellhealth.com/cannabis-menopause-symptoms-6823261.

104 Kandola, A. (2020, November 2). *Does CBD oil work for menopause symptoms?* Medical News Today. https://www.medicalnewstoday.com/articles/322078

105 Venturella, G., Ferraro, V., Cirlincione, F., & Gargano, M. L. (2021). Medicinal mushrooms: Bioactive compounds, use, and clinical trials. *International Journal of Molecular Sciences, 22*(2), 634. https://doi.org/10.3390/ijms22020634

106 Centers for Disease Control and Prevention. (2022, February). *Physical activity among adults aged 18 and over: United States, 2020* (NCHS Data Brief No. 443). U.S. Department of Health and Human Services. https://www.cdc.gov/nchs/products/databriefs/db443.htm

107 Davidson, R. (2015). Age-Related Sarcopenia. US Pharmacist, 40(5), 16–18. Retrieved April 16, 2025, from https://www.uspharmacist.com/article/agerelated-sarcopenia

108 Barker, Brenton. "Can Ice Baths Boost Testosterone? The Hormone and Libido Benefits of Cold Plunge." Recovery Guru, 26 June 2023, www.recoveryguru.com.au/blog/cold-plunge-testosterone-and-hormones/.

109 Valdez, Evelyn. "How Long To See Results From Working Out." One Fitness, 15 Jan. 2025, onefitness.com/blog/how-long-to-see-results-from-working-out.

110 Harvard Health Publishing. (2011, November). *Giving thanks can make you happier*. Harvard Medical School. https://www.health.harvard.edu/healthbeat/giving-thanks-can-make-you-happier

111 Harvard Health Publishing. (2011, November). *Giving thanks can make you happier*. Harvard Medical School. https://www.health.harvard.edu/healthbeat/giving-thanks-can-make-you-happier

112 Harvard Health Publishing. (2019, April 4). *A 20-minute nature break relieves stress*. Harvard Health. Retrieved April 24, 2025, from https://www.health.harvard.edu/mind-and-mood/a-20-minute-nature-break-relieves-stress

113 American Heart Association. (2021, March 1). *Spend time in nature to reduce stress and anxiety*. https://www.heart.org/en/healthy-living/healthy-lifestyle/stress-management/spend-time-in-nature-to-reduce-stress-and-anxiety

114 WebMD Editorial Staff. (2022, August 9). *Grounding: Benefits and techniques*. WebMD. Retrieved April 24, 2025, from https://www.webmd.com/balance/grounding-benefits

115 Singh, A., & Misra, N. (2009). Loneliness, depression and sociability in old age. *Industrial Psychiatry Journal, 18*(1), 51–55. https://doi.

org/10.4103/0972-6748.57861;:contentReference{index=1}

116 Charles, S. T., Almeida, D. M., & Mogle, J. A. (2013). Daily stressors and cortisol secretion in older adults: findings from the National Study of Daily Experiences. Psychoneuroendocrinology, 38(11), 2489–2497. https://doi.org/10.1016/j.psyneuen.2013.04.015

117 Futterman, A. D., Kemeny, M. E., Shapiro, D., & Fahey, J. L. (1994). Immunological and physiological changes associated with induced positive and negative mood. Psychosomatic Medicine, 56(6), 499–511. https://doi.org/10.1097/00006842-199411000-00005

118 "How Many Thoughts Are Negative in a Day?" Processing Therapy, 2023, https://processingtherapy.com/what-are-positive-thoughts-in-a-day/

CHAPTER 6

119 O'Connell, Julie. "Ways to Reduce Insulin Resistance for Better Blood Sugar." EatingWell, 25 Jan. 2023, https://www.eatingwell.com/ways-to-reduce-insulin-resistance-for-better-blood-sugar-8750433.

120 Telpner, Meghan. "Xenoestrogens: What Are They and Where Are They Found?" Meghan Telpner, 2023, https://www.meghantelpner.com/xenoestrogens-what-are-they-and-where-are-they-found/.

121 Kerwin, Susannah. "Visceral Fat in Menopause." Tendwell, 17 Feb. 2023, https://www.tendwellhealth.com/blog/visceral-fat-in-menopause.

122 Cleveland Clinic. (2021, August 18). *Cortisol.* https://my.clevelandclinic.org/health/articles/22187-cortisol

123 Johns Hopkins Medicine. (n.d.). *Adrenal glands.* https://www.hopkinsmedicine.org/health/conditions-and-diseases/adrenal-glands

124 Bagenstose, K. (2023, September 13). *In our blood: How the US allowed toxic chemicals to seep into our lives.* The Guardian. Retrieved April 23, 2025, from https://www.theguardian.com/environment/2023/sep/13/us-environmental-protection-agency-failed-policy-consumer-chemicals;:contentReference{index=1}

125 Hyman, Mark. "How To Reduce Your Environmental Toxin Exposure." The Doctor's Farmacy, episode 732, 9 June 2023, https://drhyman.com/blogs/content/podcast-ep732.

126   McNeilly, Claudia. "The Triumphant Return of Butter—It's Not As Unhealthy As You Think." Vogue, 14 Dec. 2016, https://www.vogue.com/article/butter-is-back-more-popular-healthy-foods.

127   Huberman, Andrew. "Dr. Mary Claire Haver: How to Navigate Menopause & Perimenopause for Maximum Health & Vitality." Huberman Lab Podcast, 3 June 2024, https://www.hubermanlab.com/episode/dr-mary-claire-haver-how-to-navigate-menopause-perimenopause-for-maximum-health-vitality.

128   Pollan, Michael. Food Rules: An Eater's Manual. Penguin Press, 2009.

129   Bellisle, France, et al. "Situational Effects on Meal Intake: A Comparison of Eating Alone and Eating with Others." Appetite, vol. 43, no. 3, 2004, pp. 269–276. doi:10.1016/j.appet.2004.06.002.

130   Blum, Dani. "The Mediterranean Diet Really Is That Good for You. Here's Why." The New York Times, 6 Jan. 2023, https://www.nytimes.com/2023/01/06/well/eat/mediterranean-diet-health.html.

131   Buettner, Dan. The Blue Zones: Lessons for Living Longer from the People Who've Lived the Longest. National Geographic Society, 2008.

132   Hyman, Mark. "The 13 Pillars of the Pegan Diet." Experience Life, 26 Feb. 2015, experiencelife.lifetime.life/article/mark-hyman-peganism.

133   Bazzano, L. A., Hu, T., Reynolds, K., Yao, L., Bunol, C., Liu, Y., . . . & Whelton, P. K. (2014). Effects of low-carbohydrate and low-fat diets: a randomized trial. *Annals of Internal Medicine*, 161(5), 309–318. https://doi.org/10.7326/M14-0180

134   Sharma, Arti, et al. "Effect of Domestic Processing on Nutritional Quality of Kidney Beans (Phaseolus vulgaris L.): A Review." Foods, vol. 12, no. 19, 2023, article 3652. PubMed Central, https://www.ncbi.nlm.nih.gov/pmc/articles/PMC10599953.

135   Harvard Health Publishing. (2021, January 1). *Time to try intermittent fasting?*. Harvard Health. Retrieved April 23, 2025, from https://www.health.harvard.edu/heart-health/time-to-try-intermittent-fasting

136   Robertson, Ruairi. "How Does Your Gut Microbiome Impact Your Overall Health?" Healthline, 3 Apr. 2023, https://www.healthline.com/nutrition/gut-microbiome-and-health.

137   Rapaport, L. (2022, July 20). *How can menopause change your gut microbiome?* Everyday Health. https://www.everydayhealth.com/menopause/how-can-menopause-change-your-gut-microbiome/

138 Wagner, M., & Oehlmann, J. (2009). Endocrine disruptors in bottled mineral water: total estrogenic burden and migration from plastic bottles. *Environmental Science and Pollution Research, 16*(3), 278–286. https://doi.org/10.1007/s11356-009-0107-7

139 Arch, Joanna J., et al. "Enjoying Food without Caloric Cost: The Impact of Brief Mindfulness on Laboratory Eating Outcomes." Behaviour Research and Therapy, vol. 79, Apr. 2016, pp. 23–34. Elsevier, doi:10.1016/j.brat.2016.02.002.

CHAPTER 7

140 Wittenberg-Cox, A. (n.d.). *Thinking*. Retrieved April 21, 2025, from https://www.avivahwittenbergcox.com/thinking

141 National Institute on Aging. (n.d.). *What is menopause?*. U.S. Department of Health and Human Services. https://www.nia.nih.gov/health/what-menopause

142 Castrillion, Caroline. 2023. "Why It's Time To Address Menopause In The Workplace." Forbes. March 22. Accessed May 7, 2024. https://www.forbes.com/sites/carolinecastrillon/2023/03/22/why-its-time-to-address-menopause-in-the-workplace/?sh=5d5d5aad1f72.

143 Faubion, S. S., Enders, F. T., Hedges, M. S., Chaudhry, R., & Kling, J. M. (2023). Impact of menopause symptoms on women in the workplace. *Mayo Clinic Proceedings, 98*(6), 409–417. https://doi.org/10.1016/j.mayocp.2023.03.021

144 Schoenberg, J., & Lautenberg, L. (2021, July 13). *Tips for women on the verge of a career change at 50*. Forbes. Retrieved April 24, 2025, from https://www.forbes.com/sites/ellevate/2021/07/13/tips-for-women-on-the-verge-of-a-career-change-at-50/

145 Oxfam Canada. (2021, April 28). *COVID-19 cost women globally over $800 billion in lost income in one year*. https://www.oxfam.ca/news/covid-19-cost-women-globally-over-800-billion-in-lost-income-in-one-year/:contentReference{index=1}

146 Lawson, M., Parvez Butt, A., Harvey, R., Sarosi, D., Coffey, C., Piaget, K., & Thekkudan, J. (2020). *Time to care: Unpaid and underpaid care work and the global inequality crisis*. Oxfam International. https://www.oxfam.org/en/research/time-care

147 UN Women & United Nations Development Programme. (2021). *From insights to action: Gender equality in the wake of COVID-19*. https://www.unwomen.org/en/digital-library/publications/2021/09/gender-equality-in-the-wake-of-covid-19

148 World Economic Forum. (2021). *Global Gender Gap Report 2021*. https://www.weforum.org/publications/global-gender-gap-report-2021/

149 National Institute on Retirement Security. (2016, March). *Women 80% more likely to be impoverished in retirement*. https://www.nirsonline.org/2016/03/women-80-more-likely-to-be-impoverished-in-retirement/

150 Wezerek, G., & Ghodsee, K. R. (2020, March 5). *Women's unpaid labor is worth $10,900,000,000,000*. The New York Times. https://www.nytimes.com/2020/03/05/opinion/women-unpaid-labor.html

151 Lepore, Jill. "The Warren Brief." The New Yorker, 21 Apr. 2014, https://www.newyorker.com/magazine/2014/04/21/the-warren-brief.

152 Jolly, S., Griffith, K. A., DeCastro, R., Stewart, A., Ubel, P., & Jagsi, R. (2014). Gender differences in time spent on parenting and domestic responsibilities by high-achieving young physician-researchers. *Annals of Internal Medicine, 160*(5), 344–353. https://doi.org/10.7326/M13-0974

153 Institute for Women's Policy Research. (2020). *Mothers' unpaid labor hours nearly double during COVID-19 pandemic*. https://iwpr.org/iwpr-issues/employment-earnings/mothers-unpaid-labor-hours-nearly-double-during-covid-19-pandemic/:contentReference{index=1}

154 Lin, I.-F., & Brown, S. L. (2021). The economic consequences of gray divorce for women and men. *The Journals of Gerontology: Series B, 76*(10), 2073–2085. https://doi.org/10.1093/geronb/gbaa157:contentReference{index=1}

155 Connell, S. (2022). *The science of getting rich for women: Your secret path to millions*. Muse Literary.

156 Albright, M. K. (2022, March 24). *Secretary Madeleine Albright on Her Legacy as a Women's Rights Champion*. Ms. Magazine. Retrieved from https://msmagazine.com/2022/03/24/secretary-madeleine-albright-women-feminist-foreign-policy/

157 Oxfam International. (2020). *Time to Care: Unpaid and Underpaid Care Work and the Global Inequality Crisis*. Retrieved from https://

policy-practice.oxfam.org/resources/time-to-care-unpaid-and-underpaid-care-work-and-the-global-inequality-crisis-620928/

158   Fidelity Investments. (2021). *2021 Women and Investing Study*. Retrieved from https://www.fidelity.com/about-fidelity/individual-investing/women-investing-study

159   NielsenIQ. (2024, April 4). *Shaping success: A deep dive into women's impact on the CPG landscape*. https://nielseniq.com/global/en/insights/analysis/2024/shaping-success-a-deep-dive-into-womens-impact-on-the-cpg-landscape/Retail Brew+3NIQ+3NIQ+3

160   Zalis, S. (2023, March 8). *The rise of the 'sheconomy'*. LinkedIn. Retrieved April 24, 2025, from https://www.linkedin.com/news/story/the-rise-of-the-sheconomy-5532977/

CHAPTER 8

161   McGinnis, D. (2018). Resilience, life events, and well-being during midlife: Examining resilience subgroups. *Journal of Adult Development*, 25(3), 198–221. https://doi.org/10.1007/s10804-018-9287-6

162   Malone, Sharon MD. (2024) Grown Woman Talk. Random House Publishing PG 301

163   Taylor, S. E., Klein, L. C., Lewis, B. P., Gruenewald, T. L., Gurung, R. A. R., & Updegraff, J. A. (2000). Biobehavioral responses to stress in females: Tend-and-befriend, not fight-or-flight. *Psychological Review*, 107(3), 411–429. https://doi.org/10.1037/0033-295X.107.3.411

164   Scharlach, A. E., & Fredriksen, K. I. (1993). Reactions to the death of a parent during midlife. *OMEGA—Journal of Death and Dying*, 27(4), 307–319. https://doi.org/10.2190/N2GW-N9WE-UEUP-9H4D

165   Monroe, V. (2023, January 15). *Val Monroe, 73: How Not to Objectify Yourself*. AGEIST. https://www.ageist.com/profile/val-monroe-73-how-not-to-objectify-yourself/

166   Shriver, M. (n.d.). *Everything Takes Time*. Maria Shriver's Sunday Paper. Retrieved April 21, 2025, from https://www.mariashriversundaypaper.com/everything-takes-time/

167   Brown, Brené. The Gifts of Imperfection: Let Go of Who You Think You're Supposed to Be and Embrace Who You Are. Hazelden Publishing, 2010.

CHAPTER 9

168 Waldinger, R. (2015). What makes a good life? Lessons from the longest study on happiness. TEDx talk. https://www.ted.com/talks/robert_waldinger_what_makes_a_good_life_lessons_from_the_longest_study_on_happiness

169 Malone, Sharon MD. (2024) Grown Woman Talk. Random House Publishing PG 287

170 Thomashauer, R. (n.d.). *Sister love for Valentine's Day?*. Mama Gena. Retrieved April 22, 2025, from https://mamagenas.com/sister-love-for-valentines/

171 Thomashauer, R. (2016). *Pussy: A reclamation* (Introduction). Hay House.

172 Aron, A., Aron, E. N., & Smollan, D. (1997). The experimental generation of interpersonal closeness: A procedure and some preliminary findings. Personality and Social Psychology Bulletin, 23(4), 363-377. https://doi.org/10.1177/0146167297234003

173 Williamson, M. (1999). *Enchanted love: The mystical power of intimate relationships* (p. 253). Simon & Schuster Paperbacks.

174 Binazir, Ali. The Tao of Dating: The Smart Woman's Guide to Being Absolutely Irresistible. Elite Communications LLC, 2013.

175 Tinx. (2023). *The Shift: Change Your Perspective, Not Yourself*. Simon & Schuster.

176 Binazir, A. (2009, July 15). *The Tao of Dating: 5 Principles to Overcome Any*. HuffPost. https://www.huffpost.com/entry/the-tao-of-dating-5-princ_b_227982

177 Wittenberg-Cox, A. (2018). *Late love: Mating in maturity*. Authors Place Press.

Books We Recommend

Anand, Margo. The *Art of Sexual Ecstasy: The Path of Sacred Sexuality for Western Lovers*. Tarcher Perigee, 1989.

Barks, Coleman. Rumi: *The Book of Love: Poems of Ecstasy and Longing*. Harper Collins, 2003.

Beattie, Melody. *Codependent No More: How to Stop Controlling Others and Start Caring for Yourself*. Spiegel and Grau, 2022.

Beattie, Melody. *Journey to the Heart: Daily Meditations on the Path to Freeing Your Soul.* Harper Collins, 1996.

Smith, Claire Bidwell LCPC. *Anxiety: The Missing Stage of Grief: A Revolutionary Approach to Understanding and Healing the Impact of Loss*. Hachette Go, 2020.

Binazir MD, MPhil., Ali. *The Tao of Dating: The Smart Women's Guide to Being Absolutely Irresistible*. Elite Communications, 2010.

Blackie, Sharon. *Hagitude: Reimagining the Second Half of Life*. New World Library, 2022.

Bluming, MD and Carol Tavris, PhD. *Estrogen Matters: Why Taking Hormones in Menopause Can Improve Women's Well-Being and Lengthen Their Lives—Without Raising the Risk of Breast Cancer*. Little, Brown Spark, 2021

Brizendine, Louanne MD, *The Female Brain*. Harmony Books, 2006.

Buettner, Dan. *The Blue Zones Kitchen: 100 Recipes to Live to 100*. National Geographic Partners, 2019.

Buettner, Dan. *The Blue Zones American Kitchen: 100 Recipes to Live to 100*. National Geographic Partners, 2022.

Casperson MD, KJ. *You Are Not Broken: Stop "Should-ing" All Over Your Sex Life*. YANB Media, 2022.

Collins, Jim. Good to Great: *Why Some Companies Make the Leap and Others Don't.* Harper Collins, 2001.

Connell, Sara. *The Science of Getting Rich for Women: Your Secret Path to Millions.* Muse Literary, 2022.

Connell. Sara. *Thought Leader Academy: 10X Your Impact and Income Through Your Mission and Message.* Muse Literary, 2023.

Dalton, Katharina and Wendy M. Hilton. *Depression After Childbirth: How to Recognize, Treat, and Prevent Postnatal Depression.* Oxford University Press, 2001.

Dr. Morse, Emily. *Smart Sex. How to Boost Your Sex IQ and Own Your Pleasure.* Park Row Books, 2023.

Dunn, Jancee. *Hot and Bothered: What No One Tells You About Menopause.* G.P. Putnam's Sons, 2023.

Fadal, Tamsen (2025). *How to Menopause: Take Charge of Your Health, Reclaim Your Life, and Feel Even Better than Before.* Hachette Go.

Frasier, Roland and Jay Abraham. *Business Wealth Without Risk: How To Create a Lifetime of Income & Wealth Every 3-5 Years.* Epic Author Publishing, 2023.

Frostrup, Mariella, and Alice Smellie, *Cracking the Menopause: While Keeping Yourself Together.* Bluebird, 2021.

Gilberg-Lenz MD, Suzanne. Menopause *Bootcamp: Optimize Your Health, Empower Your Self, and Flourish As You Age.* Harper Collins, 2022.

Gottlieb, Jen. *Be Seen: Find Your Voice. Build Your Brand. Live Your Dream.* Hay House, 2023.

Griffin, Susan. *The Book of Courtesans. A Catalogue of Their Virtues.* Broadway Books, 2001.

Gross, Rachel E., and Armando Veve. *Vagina Obscura: An Anatomical Voyage.* W.W. Norton & Company, 2023.

Haver, Mary Claire, MD, *The Galveston Diet: The Doctor-Developed, Patient-Proven Plan to Burn Fat and Tame Your Hormonal Symptoms.* Rodale Books, 2023.

Haver, Mary Claire MD, *The New Menopause: Navigating Your Path Through Hormonal Change with Purpose, Power and Facts.* Rodale Books, 2024

Hyman, Mark, MD, *Young Forever: The Secrets to Living Your Longest, Healthiest Life.* Hachette Book Group, 2023.

Kenton, Leslie. *Passage to Power: Natural Menopause Revolution*. Hay House, 1995.

Kumar MD, Rose. *Becoming Real: Reclaiming Your Health in Midlife*. Medial Press. 2014.

Lesser, Elizabeth. *Cassandra Speaks: When Women Are The Storytellers, The Human Story Changes*. Harper Collins, 2020.

Loehnen, Elise. *On Our Best Behavior: The Seven Deadly Sins and The Price Women Pay To Be Good*. The Dial Press, 2023.

Louise Hay. *You Can Heal Your Life*. Hay House, 1984.

Lundin, Mia, R.N.C., N.P. *Female Brain Gone Insane: An Emergency Guide for Women Who Feel Like They Are Falling Apart*. Health Communications, 2009.

Malone, Sharon M.D., Grown Woman Talk: Your Guide to Getting and Staying Healthy

Martin, Wednesday. *Untrue: Why Nearly Everything We Believe About Women, Lust, and Infidelity Is Wrong and How The New Science Can Set Us Free*. Little, Brown, Spark, 2018.

Mosconi PhD, Lisa. *The Menopause Brain. New Science Empowers Women to Navigate the Pivotal Transition with Knowledge and Confidence*. Avery—Penguin Random House, 2024

Mosconi PhD, Lisa. *The XX Brain: The Groundbreaking Science, Empowering Women to Maximize Cognitive Health and Prevent Alzheimer's Disease*. Penguin Random House, 2020.

Nagoski Ph.D, Emily. *Come As You Are: The Surprising Science that Will Transform Your Sex Life*. Simon & Schuster, 2015.

Northrup M.D., Christiane. *The Wisdom of Menopause: Creating Physical and Emotional Health During the Change*. Bantam Books, 2001.

Pert Ph.D, Candace B. *Molecules of Emotion: Thr Science Behind Mind-Body Medicine*. Simon & Schuster, 1997.

Pollan, Michael. *Food Rules: An Eater's Manual*. The Penguin Group, 2009.

Real, Terrence. *Us: Getting Past You & Me to Build a More Loving Relationship*. Roedale Books, 2022.

Richardson, Diana. The Heart of Tantric Sex: A Unique Guide to Love and Sexual Fulfillment. O Books, 2008.

Robbins, Tony. Diamandis, Peter, MD, Hariri, Robert MD, *Life Force: How New Breakthroughs in Precision Medicine Can Transform the Quality of Your Life & Those You Love*. Simon & Schuster, 2022.

Roman, Sanaya and Duane Parker. *Creating Money:Attracting Abundance*. HJ Kramer, Inc, 1988.

Rosensweet, Daved M.D., *Happy Healthy Hormones: How to Thrive in Menopause*. Self Published, Daved Rosensweet, 2022

Shepherd, J. (2012). *Generation M: The money, mind, and menopause connection*. BookBaby.

Silver, Tosha. *Change Me Prayers: The Hidden Power of Spiritual Surrender*. Atria—Simon & Schuster, 2015.

Sincero, Jen. *You Are A Badass At Making Money: Master The Mindset of Wealth*. Penguin Books, 2017.

Soffer, Rebecca. *The Modern Loss Handbook: An Interactive Guide to Moving Through Grief and Building Your Resilience*. Hachette Book Group, 2022.

Thomashauer, Regena. *Pussy: A Reclamation*. Hay House, 2017.

Tinx. *The Shift: Change Your Perspective, Not Yourself*. Simon & Schuster, 2023.

Turner, Teri, *No Crumbs Left: Recipes for Everyday Food Made Marvelous*. Harvest, 2019.

Urbaniak, Kasia. *Unbound: A Woman's Guide to Power*. Tarcher Perigee, 2021.

Walker, Rebecca. *Women Talk Money: Breaking the Taboo*. Simon & Schuster, 2022.

Williamson, Marianne. *A Woman's Worth*. Random House, 1993.

Williamson, Marianne. *Enchanted Love. The Mystical Power of Intimate Relationships*. Simon & Schuster, 1999.

Willson CNM, Susan. Making Sense of Menopause: *Harnessing the Power and Potency of Your Wisdom Years*. Sounds True, 2022.

Winston, Sheri CNM, RN, BSN, LMT. *Women's Anatomy of Arousal: Secret Maps to Buried Treasure*. Mango Garden Press, 2010.

Wittenberg-Cox, Avivah. *Late Love: Mating In Maturity*. Motivational Press, Inc., 2018.

ABOUT THE AUTHORS

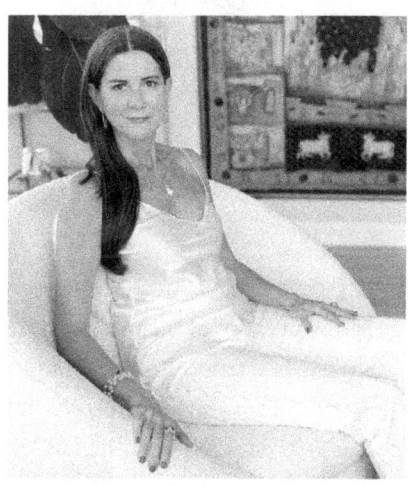

JULIE FEDELI is a devoted mother and a fierce advocate for women. While pursuing a promising career in finance, she began to practice meditation and then studied for seven years at the Barbara Brennan School of Healing and the Center for Intentional Living. But it was her complete recovery from a debilitating autoimmune illness that developed after her pregnancy that became the unlikely guide toward her true passion, helping other women become radiantly healthy and live abundantly. An inspirational entrepreneur, mentor, certified health and longevity coach, speaker, and author, Julie offers individual consulting for women longing for holistic well-being and insightful, comprehensive support for their midlife journeys. Both formally, in hosting large-scale women's events, and informally, as a maven in her community, Julie creates intentional space for women to gather in service of their highest potential. She loves delicious food, traveling to beautiful and exotic places, incredible art and music, swimming daily, and all the wonderful people in her life.

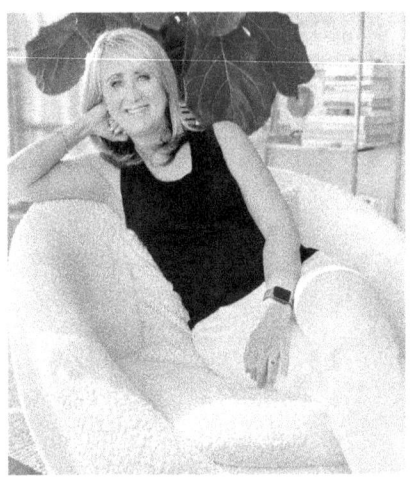

Pamela DeRose, MBA, wife and mother, tapped into the entrepreneurial drive early, accruing decades of business savvy. But it was her own midlife "crisis" that sparked her true purpose, guiding other women to harness their own inner wisdom during those chaotic years when she lacked the guidance she was looking for. Pamela graduated from the Institute for Integrative Nutrition, is a certified raw vegan chef, and a sought-after speaker. She provides practical tools to empower women to live their healthiest, most vibrant, and authentic lives through the midlife transition and beyond. When not speaking or counseling clients, you will find her in Glenview, IL, hosting family gatherings with amazing food and going for long strolls with her dear husband and rescue pup, Stella. Pamela holds space for all women ready to write their next chapter.

www.ingramcontent.com/pod-product-compliance
Lightning Source LLC
Chambersburg PA
CBHW020536030426
42337CB00013B/868